s & Answers
About Crohn's Disease
and Ulcerative Colitis:
A Lahey Clinic Guide

Andrew S. Warner, MD
Chairman of the
Department of Gastroenterology
Lahey Clinic
Burlington, MA

Amy E. Barto, MD
Department of Gastroenterology
Lahey Clinic
Burlington, MA

JONES AND BARTLETT PUBLISHERS
Sudbury, Massachusetts
BOSTON   TORONTO   LONDON   SINGAPORE

World Headquarters

Jones and Bartlett Publishers
40 Tall Pine Drive
Sudbury, MA 01776
info@jbpub.com
www.jbpub.com

Jones and Bartlett Publishers
Canada
6339 Ormindale Way
Mississauga, ON L5V 1J2
CANADA

Jones and Bartlett Publishers
International
Barb House, Barb Mews
London W6 7PA
UK

Jones and Bartlett's books and products are available through most bookstores and online booksellers. To contact Jones and Bartlett Publishers directly, call 800-832-0034, fax 978-443-8000, or visit our website at www.jbpub.com.

Substantial discounts on bulk quantities of Jones and Bartlett's publications are available to corporations, professional associations, and other qualified organizations. For details and specific discount information, contact the special sales department at Jones and Bartlett via the above contact information or send an email to specialsales@jbpub.com.

Production Credits
Executive Publisher: Christopher Davis
Production Director: Amy Rose
Associate Production Editor: Rachel Rossi
Associate Editor: Kathy Richardson
Associate Marketing Manager: Laura Kavigian
Manufacturing and Inventory Coordinator: Amy Bacus
Composition: Northeast Compositors
Cover Design: Kate Ternullo
Cover Image: © Doug Menuez/Photodisc/Getty Images, © Nick Stubbs/Shutterstock, Inc.,
© Ron Chapple/LiquidLibrary
Printing and Binding: Malloy, Inc.
Cover Printing: Malloy, Inc.

Library of Congress Cataloging-in-Publication Data
Warner, Andrew S.
    100 questions & answers about Crohn's disease and ulcerative colitis
 : a Lahey Clinic guide / Andrew S. Warner, Amy Barto.
    p. cm.
    Includes index.
    ISBN-13: 978-0-7637-3967-6
    ISBN-10: 0-7637-3967-7
    1. Crohn's disease--Miscellanea. 2. Ulcerative colitis--Miscellanea.
 I. Barto, Amy. II. Title. III. Title: One hundred questions and answers
 about Crohn's disease and ulcerative colitis.
 RC862.E52W37 2007
 616.3'44--dc22
                                                    2006015553

Printed in the United States of America
10 09 08 07 06 10 9 8 7 6 5 4 3 2

This book is dedicated to our patients.

Contents

Contents

Contents

Crohn's disease and ulcerative colitis are the two most common forms of inflammatory bowel disease (IBD). Believed to be caused by an autoimmune process, Crohn's disease and ulcerative colitis are characterized by chronic inflammation of the gastrointestinal tract, and potentially of many different organ systems throughout the body. Symptoms of inflammatory bowel disease range from mild to severe, and up to three-quarters of patients with Crohn's disease and one-third of patients with ulcerative colitis eventually need surgery. Fortunately, many effective drug therapies are currently available, with new and potentially even more effective therapies on the horizon.

100 Questions & Answers About Crohn's Disease and Ulcerative Colitis: A Lahey Clinic Guide is intended to be a patient-oriented, practical guide about Crohn's disease and ulcerative colitis. The questions are taken directly from the thousands we have been asked over the years by our patients with IBD. The answers are a compilation of the latest scientific information along with our own experience in treating inflammatory bowel disease. In essence, this book re-creates a visit to the doctor's office. It contains all the questions you wished you had asked and many that you never even thought to ask. In addition to our thoughts as physicians, two of our patients (one with Crohn's disease and one with ulcerative colitis) have also offered helpful hints and invaluable insights about living with IBD from the patient's perspective.

100 Questions & Answers About Crohn's Disease and Ulcerative Colitis: A Lahey Clinic Guide covers a wide range of issues. We explore how inflammatory bowel disease is diagnosed and treated, complications of the disease including dysplasia and cancer, when to have surgery and the different types of operations performed, diet and nutrition, lifestyle, and reproductive issues and pregnancy. This book can provide you with important and useful information, as well as an in-depth understanding of the many facets and nuances of inflammatory bowel disease.

PART ONE

The Basics

What are Crohn's disease and ulcerative colitis?

How do you get IBD?

How common are Crohn's disease and ulcerative colitis? I seem to know more and more people with it.

More ...

1. What are Crohn's disease and ulcerative colitis?

Crohn's disease and ulcerative **colitis** are the two most common forms of inflammatory bowel disease (IBD). Although the cause of IBD is unknown, it appears to be a result of disruption in the normal functioning of the **immune system**. The immune system is the body's natural defense system and works by protecting us against foreign substances that could potentially cause harm, such as viruses, bacteria, or even **cancer**. In Crohn's disease and **ulcerative colitis**, the immune system, for reasons that are not known, directs its attack against the gastrointestinal system, which is the digestive tract or tube in the body that runs from the mouth to the anus. As a result, in both diseases the intestines become chronically inflamed—red, raw, and swollen—and is often accompanied by intestinal ulcers. This ongoing **inflammation** can lead to a variety of **symptoms**, including abdominal discomfort, diarrhea, rectal bleeding, fever, and weight loss.

Both diseases cover a wide spectrum of severity. Some Crohn's disease and ulcerative colitis patients become very ill and debilitated, whereas others have symptoms that are mild and easier to control. Crohn's disease and ulcerative colitis can also affect the joints, skin, and eyes and can lead to **malabsorption** of nutrients and weight loss, **kidney stones**, **gallstones**, and many other ailments. The vast majority of individuals with Crohn's disease and ulcerative colitis need to take medication regularly, and up to 70–80% of Crohn's disease patients and 25–35% of ulcerative colitis patients eventually undergo surgery.

Colitis

inflammation of the colon; can be a result of Crohn's disease, ulcerative colitis, or other diseases.

Crohn's disease and ulcerative colitis are the two most common forms of inflammatory bowel disease (IBD). Although the cause of IBD is unknown, it appears to be a result of disruption in the normal functioning of the immune system.

Inflammation

a process characterized by swelling, warmth, redness, and/or tenderness; can occur in any organ.

Malabsorption

a condition in which the small intestine is not able to absorb nutrients and vitamins.

Jennifer's comment:

I am all too familiar with the reality of Crohn's disease. In the nearly 15 years of living with this disease, I have experienced extreme highs (symptom-free remission) and lows (debilitating pain, surgery, and recurrence) as well as everything in between. Throughout all of this, I have never allowed Crohn's disease to define who I am. Rather, it is merely an aspect of my genetic makeup that I have come to accept and learned to live with.

Crohn's disease affects different people in different ways. I can only speak to my own experiences with the disease and hope that the lessons I've learned might somehow help others who are learning to manage this unpredictable (and at times, cruel) disease.

2. What's the difference between Crohn's disease and ulcerative colitis?

From the patient's point of view, Crohn's disease and ulcerative colitis manifest with very similar symptoms. Individuals with either disorder may experience abdominal cramps, diarrhea, weight loss, intestinal bleeding, nausea, fatigue, and generalized **malaise**. To physicians, however, Crohn's disease and ulcerative colitis are quite different. Although both diseases can cause chronic and often lifelong intestinal inflammation with similar symptoms, distinguishing characteristics set them apart (see Table 1).

Crohn's disease can affect any area of the **gastrointestinal tract** from the mouth to the **anus**. Ulcerative colitis, on the other hand, is limited to the rectum and colon, never involving the small **bowel** or any other part of the gastrointestinal tract. (See Figure 1.)

*Crohn's disease can affect any area of the **gastrointestinal tract** from the mouth to the **anus**. Ulcerative colitis, on the other hand, is limited to the rectum and colon, never involving the small **bowel** or any other part of the gastrointestinal tract.*

Table 1   Characteristic Features of Crohn's Disease and Ulcerative Colitis

Characteristic	Crohn's disease	Ulcerative colitis
Site of involvement	Throughout GI tract	Colon and rectum
Pattern of involvement	Segmental disease	Continuous disease
Level of bowel wall involved	Full thickness of bowel wall	Mucosa (inside lining of bowel wall)
Granuloma cell	Present	Not present

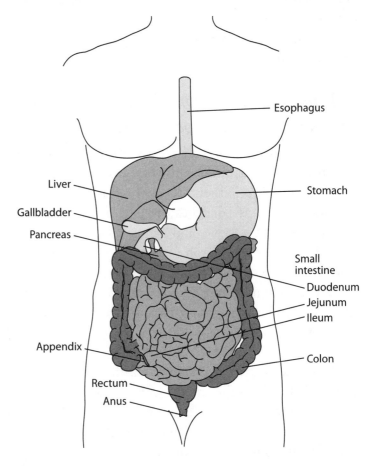

FIGURE 1 Normal gastrointestinal anatomy.

Crohn's disease may simultaneously involve different areas of the gastrointestinal tract where diseased segments of intestine alternate with normal segments; ulcerative colitis always starts in the rectum and directly extends up through the colon in a continuous and confluent fashion. Crohn's disease involves the full thickness of the bowel wall; ulcerative colitis affects only the inside lining of the rectum and colon, which is called the **mucosa**. Crohn's disease can be complicated by **fistulas** and **abscesses**, which almost never appear in ulcerative colitis. Last, in Crohn's disease on occasion a certain **cell** called a **granuloma** appears (which is why Crohn's disease, is also called **granulomatous enteritis** or **granulomatous colitis**), whereas in ulcerative colitis this particular cell is not found.

Although Crohn's disease and ulcerative colitis have many similarities and might at first glance appear to be the same disease, they are very much distinct and have distinguishing characteristics.

3. How do you get IBD?

Crohn's disease and ulcerative colitis are considered to be types of **autoimmune** diseases. Normally, the immune system functions like a defense system, guarding our bodies against attack from foreign agents—bacteria, viruses, and parasites, to name a few. An autoimmune disease occurs when the body's immune system becomes confused and starts attacking normal organs and cells, believing that they are foreign. We don't know why this happens. One theory proposes that IBD is triggered by an infection, such as a bacteria or virus, with the inflammation continuing even

Fistula

a tunnel connecting two structures that are not normally connected; examples include a fistula between the rectum and vagina (rectovaginal fistula) or the colon and bladder (colovesicular fistula).

Although Crohn's disease and ulcerative colitis have many similarities and might at first glance appear to be the same disease, they are very much distinct and have distinguishing characteristics.

Autoimmune

an inflammatory process in which your immune system attacks part of one's own body, such as the colon in ulcerative colitis.

*Crohn's disease and ulcerative colitis are considered to be types of **autoimmune** diseases.*

The Basics

Immune dysregulation

failure of the body to appropriately regulate the immune system; this lack of regulation is believed to be integral to the development of Crohn's disease and ulcerative colitis.

though the infection has long since healed. This is known as **immune dysregulation**, or a failure of the body to regulate the immune system appropriately. Many of the drugs used to control IBD focus on modulating or suppressing the immune system. Later in this book, we review this topic in detail. Also, some people have a **genetic predisposition** to develop IBD; research in this area is in its earliest stages.

If you have IBD, it is important for you to realize that you did nothing to cause yourself to develop Crohn's disease or ulcerative colitis, and you could have done nothing to prevent it. It's not from something you ate or didn't eat, it's not from drinking too much alcohol or coffee consumption, it's not from stress, it's not from working too hard, and it's not from lack of sleep. We simply do not know what causes IBD. What we do know is how to diagnose it and how to treat it.

4. Is IBD contagious?

No. Crohn's disease and ulcerative colitis are not contagious.

5. How do you know if you have Crohn's disease or ulcerative colitis?

Ulcerative colitis almost always presents with rectal bleeding or bloody diarrhea. When the inflammation is limited to the rectum, it is called **proctitis**. In patients with proctitis, red blood coating formed stool may be the only **sign** of rectal inflammation. When the inflammation extends up the left side of the colon, it is referred to as **left-sided colitis**. Inflammation that extends beyond the left side of the colon is called extensive colitis, or **pan-**

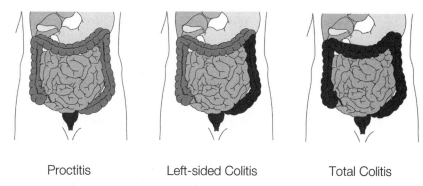

| Proctitis | Left-sided Colitis | Total Colitis |

FIGURE 2 **The three most common patterns of ulcerative colitis.**

colitis (see Figure 2). In addition to rectal bleeding, individuals with left-sided or extensive colitis also have diarrhea and lower abdominal cramps, especially when they have to move their bowels. Patients with mild ulcerative colitis have 3 to 6 loose, urgent bowel movements per day, usually accompanied by red blood. Patients with moderate ulcerative colitis will have 6 to 10 loose, urgent, bloody bowel movements per day, along with mild loss of weight and mild **anemia**. Patients with more severe ulcerative colitis can have up to 15 to 20 bloody bowel movements per day, show signs of significant weight loss, and develop more severe anemia (see Table 2). Some individuals also describe experiencing rectal spasm,

Table 2   Severity of Ulcerative Colitis

Signs and symptoms	Mild	Moderate	Severe
Frequency	3–6 BM/day	6–10 BM/day	>10 BM/day
Blood	Yes	Yes	Yes
Weight loss	No	5–10 lbs.	>10 lbs.
Anemia	No	Mild	Severe

BM, bowel movement.

7

which is called **tenesmus** and is caused by intense rectal inflammation.

Unlike ulcerative colitis, which is rather predictable in its presentation, Crohn's disease is much more varied. Therefore, Crohn's disease may be more difficult to diagnose because it can be more easily confused with other disorders. Whereas ulcerative colitis involves only the rectum, Crohn's disease can involve any area of the gastrointestinal tract and its symptoms are mostly determined by which area is affected.

Crohn's disease may be more difficult to diagnose because it can be more easily confused with other disorders.

The ileum is involved in the majority of patients with Crohn's disease, about 70% of patients (in 40% of patients the ileum alone is involved in 30% of patients, the ileum and cecum together are involved). Patients whose Crohn's disease affects this location usually present with pain in the right lower side of the abdomen, especially after eating, and often have abdominal **distention** (bloating) as well. Diarrhea and weight loss may also be seen. At times, the ileum can become narrowed to the point that the patient can develop a bowel **obstruction** (see Question 36).

Crohn's disease involves only the colon in about 20% of patients. Also called Crohn's colitis, abdominal cramps and nonbloody diarrhea are usually the presenting symptoms. While ulcers in the colon are found in both Crohn's disease and ulcerative colitis, it has never been clear why little or no rectal bleeding occurs in Crohn's colitis, whereas rectal bleeding is the predominant symptom in ulcerative colitis.

In individuals whose Crohn's disease is diffusely spread throughout the small bowel, cramps, diarrhea, and weight loss usually are the major symptoms. If the disease is severe, malabsorption accompanied by significant weight loss can also be seen. Individuals whose Crohn's disease involves the stomach and duodenum experience upper abdominal pain, nausea, and vomiting as the predominant symptoms, much as they would experience if they had an ulcer.

Sometimes it can be difficult to distinguish between Crohn's disease and ulcerative colitis. This situation may occur when Crohn's disease involves the rectum and colon and presents with symptoms much like those of ulcerative colitis. In such a case, potential ways to distinguish between the two diseases include the following:

Small bowel involvement—may be seen in Crohn's disease and is never seen in ulcerative colitis.

Appearance of ulcers on **colonoscopy**—Crohn's disease ulcers tend to be discrete and are often very deep, whereas ulcerative colitis ulcers are more confluent and superficial.

Biopsy—Crohn's disease has granulomas; ulcerative colitis does not.

Fistulas and **perianal** abscesses—can be seen in Crohn's disease and are almost never found in ulcerative colitis (see Questions 40 and 42).

Blood testing—Crohn's disease is more likely to test positive for **anti-Saccharomyces cerevisiae antibody (ASCA)**, whereas ulcerative colitis is more likely to

Sometimes it can be difficult to distinguish between Crohn's disease and ulcerative colitis.

Colonoscopy

an endoscopic procedure in which a small, thin, flexible lighted tube with a camera on the end is passed through the rectum into the colon and, at times, into the ileum; an excellent test to detect inflammation and strictures in the rectum, colon, and ileum, and one that allows for a biopsy to be taken.

Anti-Saccharomyces cerevisiae antibody (ASCA)

an antibody found in the blood that is associated with the presence of Crohn's disease.

Antineutrophil cytoplasmic antibody (ANCA)

an antibody found in the blood that is associated with the presence of ulcerative colitis.

The Basics

test positive for **antineutrophil cytoplasmic antibody (ANCA)** (see Question 8).

Ken's comment:

For me, this was a challenging diagnosis, and it was a couple of years before doctors were able to confirm I had ulcerative colitis. The first symptom I experienced was red blood coating formed stools when I had a bowel movement. When I first experienced these symptoms, I went to see my primary care physician, who referred me to a colorectal surgeon, who diagnosed ulcerative colitis. However, after a flare-up about 2 years later, I was rediagnosed by a gastroenterologist as having Crohn's. Later, further tests confirmed ulcerative colitis.

It's easy to think that these symptoms are indicative of something less serious than ulcerative colitis or Crohn's disease, and easy to not get those symptoms checked out.

I naturally had never heard of this disease before! It's important to not take even what appear to be minor symptoms lightly, and to get checked out right away. I can't express how important it is to get early and careful diagnosis and treatment for either disease, especially because they seem to manifest in people very differently. Don't be afraid to ask your doctor questions, and do as much reading and research on IBD yourself as you can.

Jennifer's comments:

Before I was diagnosed with Crohn's, neither my parents nor I had ever heard of the disease. Therefore, we had no idea what might be causing the variety of gastrointestinal "problems" I began experiencing when I was 16. Six months later, after a battery of tests and a multitude of doctor visits, we had an answer: I had Crohn's disease.

I experienced what some might consider a slow onset of Crohn's-related symptoms. My journey toward a diagnosis began with a strange taste and odor in my mouth along with a "queasy" feeling in my stomach. Although our family's dentist ruled out any obvious signs of decay or gum disease, the pain in my stomach began to worsen. Soon thereafter, my parents sought the advice of the family pediatrician, who then referred us to a gastroenterologist. At that point, I was tested for a range of disorders, including acid reflux, lactose intolerance, and a stomach ulcer. With each negative result we received back, my parents and I became increasingly frustrated; the pain I was experiencing continued to worsen and a treatment for these symptoms seemed unattainable.

At some point during those 6 months, the pain in my stomach became isolated in the lower right side of my abdomen. Eating became a dreaded activity (because the pain seemed to increase after meals), and diarrhea a daily occurrence. There were days that the pain—which made me feel like I was being stabbed repeatedly in the abdomen—was so excruciating that it was an effort just to get out of bed. All the while, my parents were forced to deal with the emotional heartache of not being able to help their child.

Relief came one morning in May 1992. After hobbling out of bed, unable to stand up straight because of the pain, my mom took me to the emergency room at a local hospital in an act of desperation. The doctors on call took one look at me and knew I was in bad shape. A few hours and an upper GI series later [see Question 8], the results were clear: I had **ileitis***, better known as Crohn's disease.*

I spent a week in the hospital "resting" my intestinal tract. This involved hooking me up to an IV and eliminating solid foods from my diet, allowing the inflammation in the affected section of my lower intestine to subside. I went home on medications, believing the worst was behind me. Nothing could have been further from the truth.

6. Can someone have Crohn's disease or ulcerative colitis and not know it?

It is not at all uncommon for someone to have Crohn's disease or ulcerative colitis without knowing it.

It is not at all uncommon for someone to have Crohn's disease or ulcerative colitis without knowing it. In fact, most IBD patients have symptoms for months to years before they seek help. In these cases, usually the symptoms are mild enough so as not to interfere with the individual's ability to go about a daily routine. For example, a man in his 60s came in to the office one day for a screening colonoscopy and was found to have classic symptoms of Crohn's disease. Upon questioning, the gentleman admitted to having loose and frequent bowel movements, about 3 to 4 a day, for more than 30 years, ever since he was a young pilot in the Vietnam War. He assumed that he had contracted an intestinal parasite, which was common in the jungle, and that he had harbored it ever since. After the war, he raised a family and had a successful career as an airline pilot without ever mentioning his bowel pattern to his physician because to him it was normal; he never felt that he was sick.

Perhaps the most famous person to have had Crohn's disease and not to have known it was President Dwight Eisenhower. In 1923, as a young Army officer, Eisenhower had an appendectomy after experiencing several episodes of pain in his right lower abdomen. For the next 33 years, Eisenhower complained of repeated episodes of lower abdominal discomfort.

Ultimately, in 1956, as President of the United States, Eisenhower had an upper GI small bowel series and was diagnosed with **regional enteritis** of the terminal ileum, which is now known as Crohn's disease. Shortly thereafter, he developed a severe bowel obstruction (see Question 36) and underwent an emergency operation where he was found to have ileal Crohn's disease, which was causing the obstruction. Rather than remove the diseased ileum, the **surgeons** bypassed the obstruction by connecting the healthy ileum above the part affected by the Crohn's disease to the healthy transverse colon below the diseased part (see Question 47). Eisenhower recovered from surgery and later that same year was elected to a second term in office. Despite having Crohn's disease for much of his adult life, Eisenhower became one of the most distinguished men of the twentieth century.

Also, people may not realize that they have IBD when their ulcerative colitis is limited to the rectum (proctitis). Individuals with proctitis often have rectal bleeding as their only symptom and mistakenly think that it is from **hemorrhoids**. Only by looking into the rectum would a physician be able to tell that the bleeding is actually from proctitis.

It is also worthwhile to point out that it is exceedingly common for young children to complain, "My tummy hurts" or "It hurts when I poop." However, such complaints usually are the way children express that they feel ill and do not suggest the start of IBD. Sometimes these types of complaints mean the child is constipated. Although it is understandable that an IBD patient who is also a parent might always be on the lookout for early signs of Crohn's disease or ulcerative

Although it is understandable that an IBD patient who is also a parent might always be on the lookout for early signs of Crohn's disease or ulcerative colitis in his or her child, it is important not to overinterpret common childhood complaints.

colitis in his or her child, it is important not to overinterpret common childhood complaints.

7. How common are Crohn's disease and ulcerative colitis? I seem to know more and more people with it.

Currently, it is estimated that approximately one million people in the United States have IBD.

Crohn's disease and ulcerative colitis are not common diseases. Currently, it is estimated that approximately 1 million people in the United States have IBD. Prior to 1960, ulcerative colitis was the more common of the two forms of IBD. Over time, however, the incidence of Crohn's disease has risen and now is nearly equal to that of ulcerative colitis. It is unclear whether this represents a true increase in numbers of people with the disease or simply better recognition of the disease. Currently, the **prevalence** (the number of people affected by a disease in a population at a specific time) of Crohn's disease and ulcerative colitis is around 75 to 150 cases per 100,000 people. IBD is more commonly found in developed countries and in northern latitudes, and is less commonly found in less industrialized countries and in more temperate climates. Also, more often IBD is seen in urban settings and is less frequently found in more rural environments.

The peak onset of Crohn's disease and ulcerative colitis usually occurs in late adolescence and extends to early adulthood (ages 15–30 years), but a person can be diagnosed with the disease at any age—from 5 to 85 years.

The peak onset of Crohn's disease and ulcerative colitis usually occurs in late adolescence and extends to early adulthood (ages 15–30 years), but a person can be diagnosed with the disease at any age—from 5 to 85 years. IBD seems to occur equally in males and females. Crohn's disease and ulcerative colitis occur more often in those of Jewish decent, with Ashkenazi Jews having the highest prevalence.

Ken's comment:

Though these are relatively uncommon diseases, I have come across several friends and acquaintances that share ulcerative colitis with me. In fact, a very close friend of mine was diagnosed with ulcerative colitis about a year after I was. It's very important to develop a support group of individuals who are going through the same challenges you are, especially when you are first diagnosed. My friend and I found solace in going out to eat together and ordering very similar meals! Because this is a very socially awkward disease, being able to empathize with individuals is a very effective way to live with the symptoms.

*Through **CCFA**, the Crohn's and Colitis Foundation of America, there are lots of resources for people with IBD who don't have a friend or relative with the disease. I'd encourage anyone to take advantage of these resources and to seek support from people going through the same medical, dietary, and social challenges you are. I'm of the mind that attitude and outlook are linked to IBD, and the more positive you can be, knowing there are others going through what you are going through, can be very helpful in managing IBD.*

Jennifer's comment:

Within a few weeks of my diagnosis, it seemed that everywhere I turned I met or learned of someone suffering from either Crohn's disease or ulcerative colitis. Although I could not ask for a more loving and supportive network of family and friends, they have never been able to relate to my disease or its effect on my physical and emotional health. The personal stories and advice I have collected from fellow Crohn's and colitis patients have had a profound impact on my ability to manage and live with my disease. Even my parents have benefited from the opportunity to speak to other parents whose children have struggled with Crohn's and colitis.

Over the years, I have encountered fellow IBD sufferers in a variety of situations and places—at school, in professional circles, through friends, at family functions, in hallways of hospitals, as well as at events sponsored by the national and local chapters of Crohn's and Colitis Foundation. I have never shied away from the opportunity to talk about my disease with others and have greatly benefited from both sharing my experiences and listening to what others have to say. In fact, it was one of my mother's colleagues at work—a colitis patient—who first introduced us to Lahey Clinic after she heard my parents were not satisfied with the care I was receiving at the time. It was there that I met Dr. Warner and have been under his care ever since (minus a few brief years in New York).

I am grateful that I have had the opportunity to interact with such a diverse group of individuals who suffer from these uncommon diseases. The realization that I was not alone in my struggles with Crohn's was incredibly therapeutic, especially in those early years.

PART TWO

Diagnosis

How are Crohn's disease and ulcerative
colitis diagnosed?

If I have Crohn's disease or ulcerative colitis,
will I pass it on to my children?

Are Crohn's disease and ulcerative colitis
ever confused with other disorders?

More ...

8. How are Crohn's disease and ulcerative colitis diagnosed?

No one test can definitively diagnose someone as having IBD with 100% certainty. Crohn's disease and ulcerative colitis are diagnosed based upon a patient's clinical history and physical examination in combination with radiologic, endoscopic, and laboratory testing. And because each patient is an individual, not all patients undergo an identical evaluation; testing is tailored to each patient. Following is a description of some of the various tests that are used in the evaluation of IBD.

No one test can definitively diagnose someone as having IBD with 100% certainty.

Radiology

- **Abdominal X ray**: Provides a picture of structures and organs in the abdomen and is helpful in detecting a bowel obstruction or **perforation**.
- **CT scan**: Uses **X rays** to create a more detailed look inside the body. A computed tomography (CT) scan is especially helpful in detecting an abscess and also is useful in evaluating for a bowel obstruction or perforation.
- **Upper GI series/upper GI series with small bowel follow-through**: Allows a close examination of the esophagus, stomach, duodenum, and small bowel. The patient must drink a thick, white liquid barium shake, and then is x-rayed as the material travels through the gastrointestinal tract. This is an excellent test to help detect **strictures**, fistulas, and inflammation in the stomach and small bowel. This test focuses specifically on the bowels, whereas a CT scan can also examine solid organs such as the liver and **pancreas**.

Upper GI series/upper GI series with small bowel follow-through

a radiologic examination of the esophagus, stomach, duodenum, and small bowel. The patient drinks a thick, white liquid shake of barium, and then the barium is tracked by taking X rays as it travels through the gastrointestinal tract. This is an excellent test to detect strictures, fistulas, and inflammation in the stomach and small bowel.

Stricture

a narrowed area of intestine usually caused by scar tissue.

- **Enteroclysis**: Provides a detailed examination of the small bowel by passing a small tube through the nose, into the stomach, and into the **duodenum**; barium is then introduced through the tube directly into the small bowel. This is an excellent test to help detect minor abnormalities in the small intestine that might not be seen on an upper GI series with small bowel follow-through.
- **Barium enema**: Allows a close examination of the rectum and colon by introducing barium through the rectum and taking X rays as it travels through the colon. This is an excellent test to help detect strictures, inflammation, and fistulas in the colon.
- **Ultrasound**: Uses sound waves to examine abdominal and pelvic organs; commonly used to look for gallstones and obstruction of the **bile duct**.
- **MRI**: uses a magnetic field to create a detailed picture of the structures and organs in the abdomen and pelvis. Magnetic resonance imaging (MRI) is especially helpful in detecting abdominal and pelvic abscesses; it can also be used to evaluate the bile duct and pancreatic duct.
- **Virtual colonoscopy**: A CT scan of the colon. This radiologic examination technique is still in the early stages of development but shows promise as a method to detect colon abnormalities.

Endoscopy

Endoscopy is a broad term that includes a variety of tests, including **upper endoscopy** and colonoscopy. Prior to a procedure, the patient receives a set of instructions describing the procedure in detail, including any preparations that may need to be made, such as stopping aspirin. All endoscopic procedures require a period of fasting beforehand. Some procedures require a colon prep, which involves flushing out the colon by way of liquid laxatives and ingestion of lots of fluids. Most but not all of these procedures are performed under **sedation**, meaning that the patient arrives early for the procedure and an IV is placed in the arm. During the procedure, intravenous sedatives are administered to the patient directly by way of the IV line (no additional needle sticks are required). These medications do not make patients completely unconscious during the procedure but rather induce a twilight state in which patients are comfortable, sleepy, and often entirely forget the procedure has happened after it is finished. Usually, patients fully wake up at the end of the procedure and ask, "When are you going to get started?"

Each of the following procedures (except **capsule endoscopy**) is performed using an endoscope (in the case of colonoscopy, the tool is called a colonoscope). An endoscope is a small, thin, flexible tube (about the width of a finger) with a light and a camera mounted on the end of the tube that is inserted through the mouth or, in the case of a colonoscope, the rectum. Endoscopes vary in length depending on the type of procedure to be performed. The physician can take a biopsy by using a set of forceps passed through a thin channel in the endoscope. The forceps removes a tiny piece of tissue that is then sent to a lab for examination under a microscope by a **pathologist**. This type of biopsy is routine and is not painful.

Potential complications of endoscopic procedures include perforation of the bowel and bleeding. These

risks are very small, and the complications are correctable. Although these procedures can be anxiety provoking, many are routine and are performed by most **gastroenterologists** on a daily basis.

Following are descriptions of the individual endoscopic procedures:

- Upper endoscopy: The endoscope is passed through the mouth into the esophagus, stomach, and duodenum. This is an excellent test to help detect inflammation and strictures in the upper gastrointestinal (GI) tract and allows for a biopsy to be taken.
- Colonoscopy: The colonoscope is passed through the rectum into the colon and, sometimes, into the ileum. This is an excellent test to detect inflammation and strictures in the rectum, colon, and ileum and allows for a biopsy to be taken.
- **Sigmoidoscopy**: This procedure is performed with or without sedation; this is a "short" version of the colonoscopy and is used to examine the rectum and the first third (left side) of the colon.
- **Proctoscopy**: This procedure is performed without sedation, usually on a special tilt table that positions the patient with his or her head down and buttocks up. In this procedure, a rigid, straight, lighted tube is used to examine the rectum. Although this procedure has mostly been replaced by flexible sigmoidoscopy, it is still an excellent test to examine the rectum.
- **Anoscopy**: This procedure is performed without sedation, usually on a special tilt table that positions the patient with his or her head down and buttocks up. In this procedure, a rigid, short, straight, lighted tube is used to examine the anal canal. This is an

Risk

the chance or probability that something will or will not happen.

Diagnosis

Proctoscopy

a procedure in which a rigid, straight, lighted tube is used to examine the rectum; usually this examination is performed on a special tilt table that positions the patient with the head down and buttocks up. Although this procedure has mostly been replaced by flexible sigmoidoscopy, it is still an excellent test to examine the rectum.

Fissure

a crack or split, which, in IBD, most often occurs in the anal canal.

excellent test to examine for an anal **fissure** or hemorrhoids.

- Enteroscopy: This procedure is performed while the patient is under sedation. A small, thin, long, flexible, lighted tube with a camera on the end, the enteroscope, is passed through the mouth into the esophagus, stomach, duodenum, and jejunum. This is an excellent test to detect inflammation and strictures in the upper GI tract and upper small intestine. This type of scope is not used very often, but it is longer than a traditional upper endoscopy scope, and thus can look deeper into the small intestine.

- Capsule endoscopy: This procedure is performed without sedation. The patient swallows a large pill (about the size of a vitamin) containing a camera and wears a sensor device on the abdomen. The capsule passes naturally through the small intestine while transmitting video images to the sensor, which stores data that can be downloaded to a computer for your physician to review. Because the capsule can travel where traditional endoscopes just can't reach, this test is mostly used in evaluating patients with chronic gastrointestinal bleeding of obscure origin. However, capsule endoscopy is not commonly used in the evaluation of Crohn's disease because other, simpler tests are usually more accurate in diagnosing and assessing the extent and severity of the disease. In addition, the capsule, which is very large, can easily become lodged in an intestinal stricture and cause an obstruction for which the patient would then need an operation to remove the capsule.

- **ERCP**: This endoscopic procedure is performed under sedation and is used to examine the bile duct and pancreatic duct. This procedure is performed for a variety of reasons, including to detect and remove stones in the bile duct, to detect **tumors** involving the bile duct and pancreatic duct, and to diagnose primary sclerosing **cholangitis**. ERCP (endoscopic retrograde cholangiopancreatography) can also be used to dilate and place stents across strictures in the bile duct and pancreatic duct (see Questions 73 and 74).

Histology

- Biopsy: Usually performed during an endoscopy. A small piece of mucosa (the inside lining of the intestine) is removed and examined under a microscope. This is an outstanding test to characterize types of inflammation and detect **dysplasia** and cancer.

Laboratory Testing

Through the use of blood tests, your physician can determine whether you are anemic, malnourished, vitamin deficient, have electrolyte imbalances, or have other abnormalities that could contribute to your symptoms. Some evidence indicates that testing positive for anti-Saccharomyces cerevisiae antibody (ASCA) suggests that a patient has Crohn's disease, and testing positive for antineutrophil cytoplasmic antibody (ANCA) suggests that a patient has ulcerative colitis. These two laboratory tests are not routine and are not usually necessary to establish a diagnosis of Crohn's disease or ulcerative colitis.

Stool Testing

Stool tests are performed to rule out an infection as the cause for intestinal symptoms. Even individuals with long-standing IBD may need occasional stool testing because an infection can arise and its symptoms can mimic those of IBD. Stool testing can also be helpful in determining causes of malabsorption.

Breath Testing

Breath testing can be performed to look for **lactose intolerance** and **bacterial overgrowth** as possible causes for your symptoms.

9. If I have Crohn's disease or ulcerative colitis, will I pass it on to my children?

Although it is true that both Crohn's disease and ulcerative colitis run in families, it is unlikely that you will pass it on to your children.

Although it is true that both Crohn's disease and ulcerative colitis run in families, it is unlikely that you will pass it on to your children. IBD is referred to as being a familial disease in that it is not uncommon for someone with IBD to have a relative, such as an aunt, uncle, or cousin, who also has Crohn's disease or ulcerative colitis. At the same time, the majority of patients with Crohn's disease and ulcerative colitis do not have children with IBD. Crohn's disease and ulcerative colitis do have a genetic basis, and the "IBD gene" runs in families, but it is not expressed in every member of the family. Why some people with the gene develop either Crohn's disease or ulcerative colitis and others don't is unclear. For this reason, there is no recommendation to perform genetic testing on a person with IBD or that person's relatives because possessing the gene does not mean that the person will actually develop Crohn's disease or ulcerative colitis. Also, there is no way to prevent IBD even if the gene is present and expressed.

10. Can I ever be cured of IBD, or will I have it for my entire life?

Unfortunately, both Crohn's disease and ulcerative colitis are chronic and usually lifelong diseases; therefore, they are diseases from which you cannot be completely cured.

Unfortunately, both Crohn's disease and ulcerative colitis are chronic and usually lifelong diseases; therefore, they are diseases from which you cannot be completely cured. Fortunately, however, both improved diagnostic capabilities and advances in treatment enable the vast majority of individuals with Crohn's disease or ulcerative colitis to be treated successfully. Patients can enjoy long periods of **remission** in which they are symptom free. From time to time, you may meet someone who states that he or she once had IBD but is now "cured" and has been free of symptoms and off medication for years—such patients are few and far between. Crohn's disease and ulcerative colitis are chronic diseases, and individuals with IBD should expect to remain on some form of long-term therapy to maintain control of their symptoms.

> **Remission**
>
> the state of having no active disease. It can refer to clinical remission, meaning no symptoms are present; endoscopic remission, meaning no disease is detected endoscopically; or histologic remission, meaning no active inflammation is detected on biopsy.

11. Can I die from having Crohn's disease or ulcerative colitis?

Although both Crohn's disease and ulcerative colitis are chronic diseases, it is exceedingly unlikely that you will die from having either one. The vast majority of patients with IBD are able to enjoy long and rewarding lives filled with work, family, friends, and leisure, no different from anyone else. Much like someone who has learned to live with the aches and pains of **arthritis**, individuals with Crohn's disease and ulcerative colitis are able to enjoy life by learning how to work around the limitations of their disease.

The vast majority of patients with IBD are able to enjoy long and rewarding lives filled with work, family, friends, and leisure, no different from anyone else.

12. Are Crohn's disease and ulcerative colitis ever confused with other disorders?

Because the symptoms of Crohn's disease and ulcerative colitis are often nonspecific and can occur in many different diseases, IBD is frequently confused with other gastrointestinal disorders. For example, diarrhea, which is one of the most common symptoms of Crohn's disease and ulcerative colitis, can occur as a result of many other intestinal disorders—infectious **gastroenteritis**, such as traveler's diarrhea or **giardiasis**; dietary causes, such as lactose intolerance or drinking too much coffee or tea; **celiac sprue**, a malabsorption disorder; an overactive thyroid; and laxative abuse. Chronic or recurrent abdominal pain may also be caused by a myriad of dysfunctions, such as gallbladder disease, **pancreatitis**, or a stomach ulcer. Rectal bleeding can occur with hemorrhoids, an anal fissure, and colon cancer. Weight loss may occur as a result of many of the conditions listed here and may also be seen with other diseases, including pancreatic cancer, **anorexia**, and **bulimia**. Last, individuals with **irritable bowel syndrome** (see Question 13) often have a combination of diarrhea and abdominal pain.

Because the symptoms of IBD are nonspecific, a physician may perform various radiologic and endoscopic tests to help make the correct diagnosis. However, sometimes even the tests do not give clear-cut answers. For example, **diverticulitis** can be confused with colonic Crohn's disease, colon cancer, or **colonic ischemia** (a condition in which the colon becomes damaged from a lack of blood flow). Infectious gastroenteritis may look almost identical to Crohn's disease or ulcerative colitis because colonic ulcers can occur in all three disorders. And because ulcers also occur in both **peptic ulcer disease** and Crohn's disease of the stomach and duodenum, these conditions can often be confused as well. Since many other diseases may mimic Crohn's disease and ulcerative colitis, physicians often order several tests to help establish a firm diagnosis.

Irritable bowel syndrome (IBS)

a functional disorder characterized by atypical abdominal pain, diarrhea, or constipation, diarrhea alternating with constipation, the feeling of incomplete fecal evacuation, or any combination of these symptoms.

Ken's comment:

*When I experienced my first major flare-up of ulcerative coli-
tis about 3 years after I was diagnosed, I had a team of doctors trying to explain the symptoms. I was tested for a variety
of allergies, infections, and other maladies because my symptoms during this flare-up were somewhat uncharacteristic of
mild ulcerative colitis. Ultimately, I was misdiagnosed with
Crohn's, and it was only after colon screening several years
later that the diagnosis was confirmed to be ulcerative colitis.
The moral of this story? Be patient. This is a tricky disease to
diagnose correctly. Listen to your doctors, ask lots of questions,
and see your doctor if your symptoms change or are unusual.*

13. Is IBD the same thing as IBS?

No. Although there is only a one-letter difference in
their names, **IBD** (inflammatory bowel disease) and
IBS (irritable bowel syndrome) are two entirely distinct and different disorders. IBD, to which this entire
book is devoted, is an intestinal disease characterized
by chronic inflammation; Crohn's disease and ulcerative colitis are the two most common forms. IBS, on
the other hand, is what is known as a functional disorder (see Table 3). A functional disorder is not a true

Table 3   Characteristics of IBS

Functional disorder
No objective abnormalities
Subjective symptoms
Atypical abdominal pain
Irregular bowel habits
• diarrhea
• constipation
• diarrhea alternating with constipation
Urgent bowel movements
Feeling of incomplete evacuation

disease but rather a collection of subjective symptoms, such as diarrhea and abdominal pain, with no actual objective abnormalities found. So, while the subjective symptoms of IBD and IBS are similar, the distinction is that with IBD, objective abnormalities are found by laboratory, radiologic, or endoscopic testing, whereas with IBS the results of all tests return normal. This is not to say that IBS is not an actual disorder or that it's just in someone's head. IBS, much like a migraine headache, does have actual, physical symptoms, but without any objective findings it cannot be classified as a disease. So, then, what is it?

IBS, as mentioned, is a functional disorder characterized by abdominal discomfort, diarrhea or constipation, sometimes diarrhea alternating with constipation, or a combination of these symptoms. Individuals with IBS are often classified as being pain-predominant, diarrhea-predominant, or constipation-predominant, depending upon the predominant symptom. The abdominal pain can be across the entire abdomen, or localized to one area of the abdomen (often the lower right or lower left side). However, some individuals with IBS may have just right upper side abdominal pain with no other symptoms. And although diarrhea is a common symptom, if one were to measure the total quantity of stool produced by someone with IBS over a 24-hour period, he or she would find that the actual stool volume was well within normal limits. So while subjectively a person with IBS may experience loose stool, the stool volume is actually normal. (Diarrhea is medically defined by stool volume and not stool consistency.) Along the same lines, individuals with constipation usually have normal **colonic transit time**, which is the amount of time it takes stool to travel

So, while the subjective symptoms of IBD and IBS are similar, the distinction is that with IBD objective abnormalities are found on laboratory, radiologic, or endoscopic testing for IBD, whereas with IBS the results of all tests return normal.

from the beginning of the colon to the rectum. (Colonic transit time is determined by a test called a stool marker study. In this relatively easy-to-perform test, the patient ingests a capsule filled with approximately 20 radio-opaque markers that can be seen on a simple abdominal X ray. If after 5 days, most of the markers are still in the colon, the patient has a delay in colonic transit. If no markers are present, the patient's colonic transit is normal. Colonic transit time is usually normal in people with IBS.)

Like IBD, IBS is a chronic disorder, and individuals with IBS learn to make appropriate lifestyle modifications. Because stress often exacerbates IBS, stress reduction is an integral part of therapy. Avoiding aggravating foods, such as fried and fatty foods, and caffeinated beverages is equally critical. If lifestyle modification alone does not control symptoms, people with IBS can take various drugs such as intestinal antispasmodics (hyoscyamine sulfate [Levsin], dicyclomine HCL [Bentyl]) as well. However, unlike IBD, the mainstay of therapy for IBS should be lifestyle and dietary modification and not pharmacologic therapy. Patients with IBS don't usually develop IBD, but patients with IBD often experience additional symptoms of IBS, which can be helped with the IBS-focused therapies mentioned here.

14. Some of my symptoms sound like those of a disease called celiac sprue. How would I know if I have this?

Celiac sprue is a malabsorption disorder that is caused by a sensitivity reaction to the protein **gluten**, which is found in wheat products such as breads and pasta. This is not a true food allergy, but an abnormal immune reaction that causes destruction of the small bowel mucosa, the intestine's innermost lining. The majority of patients with celiac sprue are completely asymptomatic; blood test abnormalities such as anemia may be the only clue to the possibility of this diagnosis. Celiac sprue and IBD share many of the same symptoms, such as diarrhea, anemia, fatigue, and weight loss. Although uncommon, patients with celiac sprue can also develop a skin rash called **dermatitis herpetiformis (DH)**. This is a very itchy, burning, stinging rash with red bumps and blisters. The rash can spread to the elbows, knees, buttocks, scalp, neck, lower back, and shoulders. Like celiac sprue, dermatitis herpetiformis can be treated with a **gluten-free diet**.

Celiac sprue runs in families and can be very common in certain parts of the world such as Ireland. Experts believe that as many as 2 million Americans may have celiac disease. However, only 3–5% who have the disease have been diagnosed. This means that the vast majority of people with celiac sprue may not have symptoms, have not sought medical attention, or have been diagnosed with something else. This disease can become active at any age. We used to think that celiac sprue was found only in very thin people, but now we know that it can be found in individuals of all body types.

A gluten-free diet is the only proven treatment for celiac sprue and to be effective, it must be strictly adhered to. Because gluten is a ubiquitous protein and is commonly found in wheat, barley, rye, and sometimes oats, this can be a formidable challenge. A nutritionist can be extremely helpful in planning healthy meal choices and in coaching you on how to avoid gluten-containing food products both at home and when eating out. If you do have celiac sprue, a gluten-free diet is the key to controlling symptoms, maintaining nutrition, and avoiding future injury to the small intestine.

Some people come to a gastroenterologist after having diagnosed themselves with celiac sprue and have experimented with their own version of a gluten-free diet. Because the symptoms of celiac sprue can be found in a variety of intestinal disorders, the diagnosis of celiac sprue cannot be made based upon symptoms alone. There are several blood tests for detecting celiac sprue, with the most accurate being an antiendomysial antibody test. This test is often combined with an upper endoscopy and a small bowel biopsy to confirm the diagnosis. A biopsy taken during an upper endoscopy is a routine and entirely painless sampling of a tiny, approximately 2- to 3-millimeter piece of small bowel mucosa. This piece of tissue is examined for signs of damage to the mucosa consistent with celiac sprue.

Celiac sprue, IBD, and many other intestinal disorders share many of the same symptoms. It is only after a thorough and complete medical evaluation that the correct diagnosis can be made. It is for this reason that individuals with intestinal symptoms should seek professional medical attention and not engage in self-diagnosis.

PART THREE

Medications

I've heard that there is a new type of prednisone with fewer side effects called budesonide (Entocort). How does it work?

What are immunomodulators and when should they be used?

What is infliximab (Remicade)?

More ...

15. Years ago my mother used to take sulfasalazine (Azulfidine) for ulcerative colitis. Is this drug still in use?

Sulfasalazine (Azulfidine) was first introduced in the 1930s to treat **rheumatoid arthritis** and was later found to be beneficial for ulcerative colitis as well. Sulfasalazine can also be used to treat Crohn's colitis. It is composed of a sulfa antibiotic in combination with an **aminosalicylate** (also known as a 5-ASA). In the colon, bacteria cleave apart sulfasalazine into the sulfa and aminosalicylate components. The sulfa half is absorbed by the body and is responsible for the majority of **side effects** associated with sulfasalazine. The aminosalicylate remains in the colon and is the active agent responsible for suppressing inflammation. Because in order to work sulfasalazine requires colonic bacteria to split it apart, its beneficial effect is mostly limited to the colon and is less helpful in small bowel disease. And because it is a sulfa-based drug, anyone with a sulfa allergy cannot take it. Even in individuals without a sulfa allergy, side effects are experienced in up to 30% of cases. Some of the more common side effects are headache, nausea, heartburn, indigestion, loss of appetite, and photosensitivity (easily burning in the sun). Less common side effects include fever, rash, muscle and joint aches, anemia, and an elevation in liver function tests. Male infertility as a result of a decrease in the sperm count may also occur; this is fully reversible within a few months of stopping the drug. (However, sulfasalazine cannot be used as a method of birth control.) Sulfasalazine is excreted by the kidneys and gives the urine a dark, yellow color, which is harmless.

Sulfasalazine is used to help control symptoms of both mild to moderate ulcerative colitis and Crohn's

Rheumatoid arthritis

a type of chronic joint inflammation.

Aminosalicylate

a class of drugs used in Crohn's disease and ulcerative colitis.

Side effect

an adverse reaction to a medication or treatment.

colitis and may take up to 3 weeks to have its full effect.

16. What are the newer sulfasalazine-type (Azulfidine) drugs used to treat Crohn's disease and ulcerative colitis?

The observation that sulfasalazine functions as a parent drug delivering the active aminosalicylate to the colon and that the sulfa component is responsible for the bulk of side effects led to the development of sulfasalazine-like drugs that are sulfa-free. In addition, these new drugs are designed to target different sites of the gastrointestinal tract. These new drugs are called aminosalicylates (see Table 4).

Like sulfasalazine, olsalazine (Dipentum) and balsalazide (Colaza) are aminosalicylates that require colonic bacteria

Table 4 Available Types of Aminosalicylates, Their Site of Action, and Usual Doses

Drug	Site of release	Usual dose
sulfasalazine (Azulfidine)	Colon	1 g two to four times daily
olsalazine sodium (Dipentum)	Colon	500 mg two to three times daily
balsalazide disodium (Colazal)	Colon	2.25 grams three times daily
mesalamine (Asacol)	Ileum and colon	800–1600 mg two to four times daily
mesalamine CR (Pentasa)	Small bowel and colon	1 g three to four times daily

to activate them and, therefore, target the colon. They have limited effectiveness in the small bowel. Mesalamine (Asacol) and mesalamine CR (Pentasa), on the other hand, are aminosalicylates that target the small bowel as well as the colon. Mesalamine is released in the lower small bowel, called the ileum, whereas mesalamine CR is released throughout the small intestine. Although fewer side effects have been observed with these newer aminosalicylates than with sulfasalazine, patients may still experience intestinal discomfort, loose stool, indigestion, and rash. Some individuals who use mesalamine and mesalamine CR experience hair loss. Diarrhea, caused by an increase in fluid secretion by the small bowel, has been described in patients taking olsalazine (Dipentum); this usually subsides within a few days. In a number of reports, pancreatitis is associated with use of the aminosalicylates. Male infertility, which is a common side effect of sulfasalazine, has not been described in association with these drugs.

Because osalazine and balsalazide disodium target the colon, like sulfasalazine, they are used for mild to moderate ulcerative colitis and Crohn's colitis. Mesalamine and mesalamine CR, which are released in the small bowel, are often prescribed for patients with small bowel Crohn's disease, in addition to those whose Crohn's disease involves the colon and those who have ulcerative colitis. The aminosalicylates take approximately 3 weeks before they are fully effective.

17. What is the role of topical therapy in treating proctitis, and is topical therapy used for treating anything else?

Topical therapy is therapy in which you apply medicine directly to the tissue, much like when you apply medicated ointment to a skin rash. Individuals with IBD, especially ulcerative colitis, can be thought of as having a rash of the colon. As for the skin, applying medication directly to the inflamed tissue can be extremely effective.

For example, an elderly professor who has had ulcerative colitis since the 1950s mentioned one day that for many years, whenever he had an ulcerative colitis flare, he would break apart his sulfasalazine capsules and place them directly inside his rectum. He believed that doing this helped quiet down the flare. On his own, the professor had discovered the benefits of topical therapy.

Topical therapy applied rectally comes in four preparations (see Table 5): creams and ointments (Analpram, Proctocream), which are used around and inside the anus; suppositories (Anusol, mesalamine [Canasa]), which are placed directly inside the rectum; foam (hydrocortisone acetate [Cortifoam], Proctofoam),

Individuals with IBD, especially ulcerative colitis, can be thought of as having a rash of the colon.

Table 5   Topical Preparations, Their Site of Action, and Indications for Use

Topical preparation	Site of action	Indications
Creams and ointments	Around and in the anus	Anal fissure, perianal dermatitis
Suppository	Rectum	Proctitis
Foam	Rectum and lower sigmoid colon	Proctitis and proctosigmoiditis
Enema	Rectum and left colon	Left-sided colitis

which is squirted into the rectum and can travel up as high as the lower sigmoid colon; and enemas ([hydrocortisone enema] Cortenema, mesalamine [Rowasa]), which are squirted into the rectum and can travel up the entire left colon. **Corticosteroids** come in all four preparations, whereas mesalamine comes as a suppository and as an enema.

Corticosteroid

a potent anti-inflammatory drug.

Corticosteroid creams and ointments are used mostly for anal fissures and inflammation around the anus (perianal **dermatitis**). Suppositories are used for individuals with proctitis (rectal inflammation). The foam preparation is also used for proctitis, as well as **proctosigmoiditis** (inflammation of the rectum and lower sigmoid colon). Enemas are used for left-sided colitis. All four preparations can be used either alone or in combination with oral medication.

Dermatitis

skin irritation or inflammation; in IBD it often occurs around the anus.

Proctosigmoiditis

inflammation of the rectum and sigmoid colon.

Topical therapy is frequently used to treat proctitis. Individuals with proctitis often describe a variety of symptoms—red blood coating the stool, or passing clots of red blood; frequent urges to have a bowel movement; intense rectal spasm; and/or little to no diarrhea. These symptoms can occur from once or twice a year, to once or twice a day. Individuals who have infrequent episodes of proctitis can often be treated with topical therapy when they have symptoms and need not take any medication when they are feeling well. Individuals who suffer from daily symptoms, on the other hand, need to use topical therapy on a more regular basis. For example, while some patients must take a daily suppository to control their symptoms, others can use a suppository every other day or every third day. Individuals with daily symptoms of proctitis are often prescribed a combination of oral medication, such as an aminosalicylate, along with topical therapy to achieve the best results. Most individuals with proctitis experience symptoms on and off for many years. Fortunately, only 15% to 25% of individuals with proctitis progress to having ulcerative colitis, with the remainder staying as proctitis.

Topical therapy is also often used to treat ulcerative colitis. When enemas are used for left-sided colitis, they are usually given in addition to oral therapy, although in some cases they may be used alone. Treatment of anal fissures and perianal dermatitis are covered in Questions 41 and 44, respectively.

18. I've heard that prednisone is commonly used to treat Crohn's disease and ulcerative colitis. When should you use prednisone, what are its side effects, and is it safe?

Corticosteroids are one of the mainstays of therapy for IBD. First used to treat active ulcerative colitis in the 1940s, they were later found to be helpful in Crohn's disease as well. Prednisone is the corticosteroid most commonly prescribed and is used most often in individuals with moderately to severely active Crohn's disease and ulcerative colitis. Although these patients often are first treated with a less potent drug, such as an aminosalicylate, this is not required. In the appropriate setting, prednisone can be used as first-line therapy. When to start prednisone depends upon the severity of the symptoms and the physician's and patient's preferences.

Corticosteroids are one of the mainstays of therapy for IBD.

*Prednisone has clearly been demonstrated to be effective for **induction of remission**, but it has not been shown to be beneficial in **maintenance of remission**.*

Prednisone is usually dosed at 40 to 60 milligrams (mg) daily, either as a single dose in the morning or in divided doses (taken after breakfast and after dinner, for example). It usually starts working within 1 to 2 weeks. Prednisone has clearly been demonstrated to be effective for **induction of remission**, but it has not been shown to be beneficial in **maintenance of remission**. In other words, prednisone is good at treating the acute symptoms of active Crohn's disease and ulcerative colitis, but it is not helpful as long-term therapy.

How long a patient can safely be on prednisone is a subject of much debate. Usually, the duration of therapy is from a few weeks to a few months. Prednisone should never be abruptly discontinued but rather slowly tapered off, commonly by 5 to 10 milligrams each week. Abrupt discontinuation can be potentially life-threatening by inducing a sudden drop in blood pressure, which is also known as an **adrenal crisis**. When you take prednisone, your adrenal glands become dormant and stop producing cortisone, the body's own natural corticosteroid. Among other things, cortisone is responsible for maintaining a stable blood pressure. Slowly tapering off use of prednisone enables the adrenal glands to wake up and restart cortisone production. However, if prednisone is abruptly discontinued, the adrenal glands are caught by surprise and are unable to quickly make enough cortisone to support an adequate blood pressure.

Even patients who slowly taper prednisone can develop the **prednisone-withdrawal syndrome** (also called **steroid withdrawal syndrome**), which is characterized by fatigue, lethargy, lassitude, and muscle and joint aches. These symptoms may last up to 5 weeks. The only effective treatment is for the patient to go back on prednisone with an even slower taper. Some patients, however, prefer to wait out the withdrawal symptoms rather than restart prednisone.

Unfortunately, prednisone use is commonly associated with a multitude of side effects, although not every individual who takes prednisone experiences these side effects. Early side effects include insomnia, mood swings, tremulousness, acne, fluid retention, a voracious appetite, weight gain, and hyperglycemia. **Diabetes**, **hypertension**, **cataracts**, **osteonecrosis** of the hip, and **osteoporosis** have been observed with longer-term use.

Because of these **adverse effects** from prednisone, as well as its lack of long-term effectiveness, patients and physicians alike are often reluctant to use prednisone. Nonetheless, prednisone remains an effective agent in the treatment of IBD and, when employed appropriately, can provide rapid relief from often debilitating symptoms. The goal is to use corticosteroids to control a flare and then taper them as quickly but safely as possible. Corticosteroids can be both a blessing and a curse.

Jennifer's comment:

I was prescribed prednisone immediately following my diagnosis. My family and I likened it to my miracle drug—it provided me with immediate relief from the debilitating pain I was experiencing. On prednisone, after

Medications

Diabetes
elevated blood sugar (glucose).

Hypertension
high blood pressure.

Cataracts
a clouding of the eyes' natural lens; occurs naturally with age, but their development can be accelerated with chronic use of corticosteroids.

Osteonecrosis
also called avascular necrosis; severe deterioration of the bone. It can occur after long-term use of corticosteroids and is usually diagnosed by an MRI of the affected joint.

Osteoporosis
a severe decrease in bone density; can occur after long-term use of corticosteroids.

Adverse effect
side effect to a medication or treatment.

months of unbearable suffering, I began to feel like my old self again.

I was on and off prednisone the year following my diagnosis as a result of ongoing, acute flare-ups. Unfortunately, despite the reprieve the medication provided me from my symptoms, I fell victim to its nasty side effects. By the time I came under Dr. Warner's care, I had developed some obvious signs of a prednisone user—I had gained a substantial amount of weight as well as what some physicians and patients often refer to as moon cheeks—a rounding of the cheeks. People I knew even commented on my "chipmunk" cheeks to my face (and behind my back, I'm sure). I also experienced moderate mood swings that came on with absolutely no warning.

I was 17 at the time, and the combination of these side effects were particularly difficult for me to handle. I clearly remember trying to convince Dr. Warner to aggressively wean me off the drug in the weeks preceding my senior prom (I believe I actually suggested that I stop the drug altogether). Needless to say, I was unsuccessful in my negotiations. Although I know that prednisone played a critical role in the early treatment of my disease, the side effects became too much for me to bear. In fact, I still have difficulty looking at my prom and graduation pictures. They are a painful reminder of my experiences with Crohn's disease that year.

Despite the fact prednisone proved an effective short-term treatment for my disease, I came to despise the drug. To this day I would avoid taking prednisone at all costs. For me, the physical and psychological impact of the drug far outweighs the benefits.

19. I've heard that there is a new type of prednisone with fewer side effects called budesonide (Entocort). How does it work?

Budesonide (Entocort) is a corticosteroid that is approved for use in mild to moderately active Crohn's disease involving the ileum and right colon. Budesonide is released and becomes highly concentrated in the ileum, which is why it is believed to be effective for Crohn's disease affecting this area. Because it is absorbed into the bloodstream much less than prednisone, and is rapidly metabolized by the liver, budesonide has fewer and less intense corticosteroid-type side effects. The typical prednisone side effects, such as insomnia, mood swings, and jitteriness, may still occur. But they are seen less frequently and are usually not as severe. The effect of budesonide on the development of osteoporosis is still being studied.

Who should use budesonide instead of prednisone? Budesonide is appropriate for individuals who need to go on prednisone but previously found its side effects to be severe and intolerable, or for those who need to go on prednisone and are anxious about the side effects. Budesonide is nearly as effective as prednisone but has a slower onset of action.

Budesonide comes as 3-milligram tablets and is usually dosed at 9 milligrams (three tablets) daily for roughly 4 weeks, and then is tapered to 6 milligrams daily for 2 weeks, 3 milligrams daily for 2 weeks, and then stopped. However, physicians often modify this regimen based upon an individual's symptoms and response to therapy. Like prednisone, budesonide is

Because it is absorbed into the bloodstream much less than prednisone, and is rapidly metabolized by the liver, budesonide has fewer and less intense corticosteroid-type side effects.

Medications

used for control of acute symptoms and has not been demonstrated to be an effective drug for long-term therapy of Crohn's disease. Budesonide has not been approved for use in ulcerative colitis, although some physicians prescribe it in place of prednisone for ulcerative colitis as well as for other diseases.

20. What are immunomodulators and when should they be used?

Immune modulators

a class of drugs that modulates or suppresses the immune system.

Azathioprine (Imuran) and 6-mercaptopurine (6-MP) are the two **immune modulators** most commonly prescribed in the treatment of IBD. Azathioprine is converted in the liver to 6-MP; the drugs are considered interchangeable, although the dosing is different. These drugs are usually given to patients with Crohn's disease and ulcerative colitis who respond to prednisone but flare every time prednisone is withdrawn (known as being prednisone dependent) or patients who continue to have active symptoms despite being on an adequate dose of prednisone (known as being prednisone refractory). In addition to being helpful in treating active symptoms, azathioprine and 6-MP have also been shown to be effective in maintaining remission and, as a result, are used for long-term therapy. Some evidence suggests that azathioprine and 6-MP may be helpful for treating fistula disease. Often, azathioprine and 6-MP are given concomitantly with infliximab (Remicade) to reduce the likelihood of developing an allergic reaction (see Question 21).

In addition to being helpful in treating active symptoms, azathioprine and 6-MP have also been shown to be effective in maintaining remission and, as a result, are used for long-term therapy.

Although many patients are concerned about using drugs that modulate or suppress their immune system, azathioprine and 6-MP are usually very well tolerated. One of the potential adverse reactions includes bone marrow suppression. This can be seen in approximately 2% of patients and can lead to a lowered white blood count, anemia, and/or a low platelet count. For this reason, people who take azathioprine or 6-MP should be carefully monitored and must have their complete blood count checked on a regular basis—usually weekly for 1 month, monthly for about 6 months, and then approximately every 3 to 6 months. Patients should also be monitored for elevation in the liver function tests. Both bone marrow suppression and rising liver function tests are reversible by decreasing the dose of these drugs or stopping them entirely. Individuals taking azathioprine or 6-MP are also more prone to infection, especially if the white blood count is suppressed to an unacceptably low level.

Pancreatitis, which is inflammation of the pancreas, is an allergic reaction to azathioprine or 6-MP and, if it occurs, usually happens within 1 month of starting the medication. Seen in approximately 2% of IBD patients taking azathioprine or 6-MP, the symptoms of pancreatitis include severe upper abdominal pain, nausea, vomiting, and fever. The diagnosis of pancreatitis can be confirmed when the results of a blood test show a rise in the levels or amylase and lipase, which indicates pancreatic inflammation, and by a CT scan of the abdomen that reveals an inflamed pancreas.

Other side effects of azathioprine and 6-MP include nausea, fever, and muscle and joint aches. There have also been rare reports of **lymphoma** in individuals taking azathioprine or 6-MP.

Lymphoma
cancer of the lymphatic system, that is, the lymph nodes.

Azathioprine and 6-MP are dosed based on your body weight—azathioprine is dosed at 2 to 2.5 milligrams per kilogram of body weight, and 6-MP is dosed at 1.5 to 2 milligrams per kilogram of body weight. The main downside of azathioprine and 6-MP is that it may take between 2 and 6 months to reach their full effect, although some patients respond more quickly. The rate of response likely depends on the dose you start with; if you start by taking a higher dose, you'll experience a faster response. The differing response rate between individuals may also be because the individual rate of enzymatic breakdown of azathioprine and 6-MP by an enzyme called TPMT. Eighty-nine percent of the population has a normal level of TPMT and should be started at a normal dose of Imuran or 6-MP; 10% to 11% of the population has a below-normal level of TPMT and should be started on a lower-than-usual dose; 0.3% of the population has no detectable level of this enzyme. It is not considered safe for those without any detectable enzyme to take azathioprine or 6-MP because the drugs cannot be broken down and severe toxicity would likely ensue. For this reason, if you are placed on azathioprine and 6-MP, you should first have your TPMT enzyme level checked (which is done with a blood test).

Some literature suggests that azathioprine and 6-MP should be dosed by measuring the enzymatic breakdown products of azathioprine and 6-MP, which are known as 6-MP metabolites, instead of dosing azathioprine and 6-MP based on your weight. Although the concept of dosing these drugs to achieve a certain blood level is appealing, scientific evidence to support this approach is limited. This is a hot topic among physicians who treat IBD. In time, more data will become available to settle this controversy.

Jennifer's comment:

I have been prescribed azathioprine and 6-MP at different times over the years, and have had very different experiences with both medications. Although routine blood tests never revealed any abnormalities with my liver or bone marrow counts, it seems that azathioprine had a more severe impact on my immune system than 6-MP did.

While on azathioprine I contracted the chicken pox for the first time at the ripe age of 18. Soon after those dreaded spots made their ugly debut on my body, I began experiencing sharp pains in my lower back. Dr. Warner did not hesitate to hospitalize me (much to my dismay) for intravenous therapy to prevent the chicken pox virus from spreading. (Author's note: While chicken pox is usually a mild childhood illness, in a person who is immunocompromised it can become life threatening.) My azathioprine was immediately discontinued, and after a few very uncomfortable days in a hospital bed, I was sent home to itch my way back to normal health.

In contrast, I have been on 6-MP for nearly 6 years in an effort to maintain my remission and have been in exceptionally good health the entire time. In fact, I have not experienced any difficulty fighting off occasional colds or viruses while on the drug. Despite these positive indicators, I continue to get routine blood tests (every 3 months) as well as an annual flu shot to decrease my chances of a prolonged illness while on 6-MP. However, I am hopeful that this long-term therapy is effectively prolonging my remission.

21. What is infliximab (Remicade)?

One of the most significant advances in the treatment of IBD, infliximab (Remicade) has proved itself effective for use in both Crohn's disease and ulcerative colitis, as well as in other ailments, such as rheumatoid arthritis. Infliximab is used to treat active symptoms of IBD in patients who do not respond to conventional therapy and as a maintenance drug for patients in remission. Initially, infliximab was used mostly for individuals with severe symptoms who did not respond to prednisone and/or immunomodulating agents. More recently, infliximab is being introduced earlier as an alternative to corticosteroids in patients with milder symptoms. Some physicians advocate using infliximab as initial therapy for IBD without first attempting treatment using the more traditional approach. Although from time to time this may be appropriate, infliximab is still used predominately for individuals who are refractory to conventional therapy.

One of the most significant advances in the treatment of IBD, infliximab (Remicade) has proved itself effective for use in both Crohn's disease and ulcerative colitis, as well as in other ailments, such as rheumatoid arthritis.

Infliximab is a part-human, part-mouse antibody that is administered as an IV infusion. It's designed to attack a protein in the immune system called TNF-alpha, which plays a critical role in the initiation of the inflammatory process in IBD. By targeting TNF-alpha, infliximab is able to suppress and prevent the inflammation that is the hallmark of IBD. **TNF** stands for *tumor necrosis factor*. TNF was first found in the setting of tumors. We now know that TNF is a protein that is commonly found in many inflammatory conditions and does not indicate that someone has a tumor. Unfortunately, the name has stuck.

TNF

tumor necrosis factor; this protein plays a central role in the initiation of inflammation in IBD. First described in the setting of tumors, we now know that TNF is commonly found in many inflammatory conditions.

Infliximab is usually given as three IV infusions over a 6-week period, followed by an infusion every 8 weeks.

It works rapidly, and most patients experience significant improvement in their symptoms within 2 weeks after the infusion; some patients feel better in just 1 or 2 days. The usual dose of infliximab is 5 milligrams per kilogram of body weight. Not uncommonly, after taking infliximab for a while, some patients start having IBD symptoms before the next scheduled infusion. In these cases, patients can take infliximab more frequently (e.g., every 6 weeks), or the dose can be increased to 10 milligrams per kilogram of body weight.

Infliximab is generally well tolerated. One of the most common side effects is the development of an allergic reaction to infliximab. When you have an allergic reaction, it is usually after multiple infliximab infusions; it is unusual for you to have an allergic reaction during the initial infusion. Allergic reactions are more likely to occur if the interval between infliximab infusions is longer than recommended. In other words, if you receive infliximab infusions every 8 weeks as maintenance therapy, you are less likely to develop an allergic reaction than is someone who receives a infliximab infusion less frequently, such as every few months.

Infliximab (Remicade) is generally well tolerated.

Why would you want to get infliximab less frequently than recommended? Some patients, as well as some physicians, believe that infliximab should be given only at the time of a flare. This is called episodic therapy. When you receive infliximab episodically you are more likely to develop **antibodies to infliximab**, or **ATIs** and, as a result, are more likely to experience an allergic reaction than is someone who receives infliximab as part of a regularly scheduled maintenance program. You might develop antibodies to infliximab

Antibodies to infliximab (ATIs)

because infliximab (Remicade) is partially derived from mouse cells, the immune system detects that Remicade is foreign and creates these antibodies to fight against it.

because infliximab is partially derived from mouse cells, and your immune system may recognize it as a foreign substance and create antibodies to attack it.

For individuals receiving infliximab episodically, taking azathioprine or 6-mercaptopurine (6-MP) concomitantly reduces the likelihood of developing antibodies to infliximab; as a result, these individuals experience fewer allergic reactions. Giving these individuals a corticosteroid immediately prior to the infusion may also reduce the risk. Both of these measures have also been shown to reduce the likelihood of developing antibodies to infliximab in individuals who receive regularly scheduled maintenance infliximab infusions. However, because those receiving maintenance therapy are much less likely to develop antibodies, it is not as critical that they take measures to help mitigate against antibody development.

Most allergic reactions to infliximab are mild and can be treated by slowing down the rate of infusion. Taking acetaminophen (Tylenol) and diphenhydramine (Benadryl) can also be helpful. The types of mild reactions commonly experienced include flushing, difficulty catching your breath, chest heaviness, lightheadedness, headache, and muscle and joint aches. If you develop an allergic reaction, on subsequent infusions you should take acetaminophen and diphenhydramine, and sometimes IV hydrocortisone, immediately prior to receiving infliximab. True anaphylactic reactions—hives, wheezing, drop in blood pressure—are not as common. If they do occur, infliximab should be stopped immediately and you should be treated with IV diphenhydramine, IV hydrocortisone, and, if severe, epinephrine. If you develop an anaphylactic reaction to infliximab, you are at significant risk for having a severe and potentially life-threatening reaction with further exposure to the drug. Therefore, a careful risk-benefit assessment must be made before you consider any further therapy with infliximab.

Individuals receiving infliximab also have a higher rate of infections. Common cold symptoms can be seen in up to 25% of patients. These usually resolve within a week. More serious infections are less common, occurring in approximately 3% of patients. One of the most serious infections is active **tuberculosis**. Infliximab does not cause tuberculosis; however, infliximab can reactivate **latent tuberculosis** that might have been contracted years earlier. Infliximab should never be used in any patient with untreated or inadequately treated tuberculosis. All patients who are candidates for infliximab must have a negative skin test for tuberculosis prior to starting therapy. Patients who potentially could have been exposed to tuberculosis previously should also have a chest X ray. Currently, no recommendation exists for follow-up testing for tuberculosis exposure after you have started infliximab. You should be advised to avoid traveling to an area of the world where tuberculosis is common. If you may have been exposed to tuberculosis after starting infliximab, no additional infusions should be given until tests prove you have not contracted tuberculosis. If you do contract tuberculosis, you need to be under treatment for active tuberculosis before receiving any further therapy with infliximab.

Infliximab should not be used in individuals with untreated congestive heart failure and should be used with caution if you have a history of liver disease or blood or neurological disorders.

Tuberculosis

an infection with *Mycobacterium tuberculosis.*

There have been rare reports of lymphoma and malignancy in patients receiving infliximab. Most recently, an aggressive type of lymphoma, called hepatosplenic T-cell lymphoma, has been reported in young patients on concomitant infliximab with azathioprine or 6-MP. There have been no reported cases of this type of lymphoma in patients taking infliximab alone.

22. What is the role of cyclosporine in IBD?

Cyclosporine is a potent immunosuppressive drug that has revolutionized organ transplantation. Prior to the advent of cyclosporine, transplant recipients frequently died as a result of their bodies' immune systems attacking the transplanted organs. By suppressing the transplant recipient's immune system, cyclosporine has been able to improve an individual's ability to live without rejecting his or her new organ. Because in ulcerative colitis the immune system appears to attack the colon, it was theorized that cyclosporine could be similarly beneficial in mitigating this autoimmune response. In the early 1990s, this theory was in fact found to be true. In more than 80% of hospitalized ulcerative colitis patients who had severe symptoms despite being on IV corticosteroids and who were at risk for a **colectomy** (surgical removal of the colon), cyclosporine dramatically and rapidly improved symptoms. As a result of this finding, cyclosporine is now used as an alternative to colectomy in hospitalized, **steroid-refractory** ulcerative colitis patients.

Cyclosporine has two main downsides that limit its usefulness. First, cyclosporine is effective for only a few months, after which most patients have a flare of their

In more than 80% of hospitalized ulcerative colitis patients who had severe symptoms despite being on IV corticosteroids and who were at risk for a colectomy (surgical removal of the colon), cyclosporine dramatically and rapidly improved symptoms.

Steroid-refractory

a term used to describe an individual who does not have symptomatic improvement with use of a corticosteroid.

symptoms. Accordingly, cyclosporine is used as a bridge either to longer-term immune-modulating therapy with azathioprine or 6-mercaptopurine (6-MP) or to elective colectomy. Second, cyclosporine is a potent drug with significant potential side effects. These include anaphy-lactic shock, hypertension, severe infections, kidney insufficiency, abnormal liver function tests, seizures, nerve damage, and excess hair growth. And although most of these problems are reversible when the dose is decreased or discontinued, sometimes permanent dam-age occurs. Therefore, individuals on cyclosporine must be carefully and closely monitored through frequent office visits and laboratory testing. In addition, the majority of patients are also concomitantly placed on antibiotics to help ward off a potentially lethal lung infection called *Pneumocystis carini* pneumonia, or PCP.

Should every hospitalized ulcerative colitis patient who does not respond to IV corticosteroids be placed on cyclosporine? Given its limited duration of action and potential severe side effects—no. Cyclosporine should be viewed as one part of the armamentarium to com-bat severe ulcerative colitis; it is not the most appropri-ate treatment for every patient. As with any therapy, and more so with a drug that has potentially serious side effects, the benefits have to be weighed against the risks. For a young, otherwise healthy patient recently diagnosed with ulcerative colitis who is suddenly fac-ing the urgent need for a colectomy, cyclosporine may be a good option to allow more time for the person to learn about and accept this new diagnosis. On the other hand, an older patient who has had chronic ulcerative colitis for many years may more readily accept the need for surgery and may be physiologically less tolerant of any potential side effects of the drug.

Cyclosporine has little role in the treatment of Crohn's disease. A few small studies show benefit for patients with fistulizing Crohn's disease. Infliximab has now largely supplanted this indication.

Cyclosporine is a rapidly acting and potent immuno-suppressive agent that has many potentially serious side effects. It should be administered only in hospitals and by physicians experienced in using it to treat severe ulcerative colitis.

23. What is the role of methotrexate?

For many years, methotrexate has been used in the treatment of rheumatoid arthritis and **psoriasis**. Some evidence suggests that it may be helpful for Crohn's disease as well. In a 16-week trial comparing weekly injections of methotrexate to placebo in patients with active Crohn's disease despite being treated with pred-nisone, 39% of patients who took methotrexate went into remission as compared to 19% of patients who received placebo. Those patients who achieved remis-sion were then given either weekly injections of methotrexate or a placebo for an additional 40 weeks. Sixty-five percent of those receiving methotrexate remained in remission at the conclusion of the 40-week trial, as compared with 39% of those on placebo.

Although results of both of these trials were statisti-cally significant (which means the results are probably true and not caused by chance), methotrexate has never really caught on as a major therapy for Crohn's disease. This is most likely because even though the trials reached **statistical significance**, only a minority of patients achieved remission. In addition, methotrex-

Psoriasis

a type of chronic skin inflammation.

In a 16-week trial compar-ing weekly injections of methotrexate to placebo in patients with active Crohn's disease despite begin treated with predni-sone, 39% of patients who took methotrexate went into remission as compared to 19% of patients who received placebo.

Statistical significance

a term that means the results reported in a scientific study (i.e., an experiment) are probably true and did not occur by chance.

ate also has a number of potentially serious adverse effects. It can cause liver damage, including **liver fibrosis** and **cirrhosis**, and, therefore, should not be given to individuals with preexisting liver disease. As a result, some patients who take methotrexate must undergo periodic liver biopsies to assess whether any damage to the liver has occurred. Methotrexate can also cause toxicity to the lungs and bone marrow. Methotrexate is listed by the FDA as category x, meaning that it is known to cause birth defects. Methotrexate can affect the baby both when the woman is treated and the man is treated. Therefore, Methotrexate should not be used during pregnancy. Both partners should stop the drug at least 3 months prior to planned conception. Other common side effects include nausea, hair loss, headache, dizziness, drowsiness, and mouth sores. And because methotrexate reduces the absorption of folic acid, all patients should take supplemental folic acid tablets.

Liver fibrosis
scar tissue in the liver, usually from prior inflammation.

Cirrhosis
a condition in which the liver has become severely scarred; most commonly caused by excess alcohol use or viral infection, but can also be a result of medication.

Adjunctive therapy
using a drug or therapy in addition to the primary therapy.

24. What is the role of antibiotics in Crohn's disease?

The role of antibiotics as primary and **adjunctive therapy** (using antibiotics in addition to the primary drug) is one of the most controversial issues in the treatment of Crohn's disease. Even though only a paucity of evidence supports their use, many physicians strongly believe that antibiotics provide a true benefit. Although only a few randomized controlled trials demonstrate clear-cut efficacy, clinical experience has led to their routine use.

If antibiotics are, in fact, beneficial in Crohn's disease, it is unclear why they are. One theory holds that if

The role of antibiotics as primary and adjunctive therapy (using antibiotics in addition to the primary drug) is one of the most controversial issues in the treatment of Crohn's disease.

Medications

antibiotics do work, it is because they treat an undiagnosed bacterial infection and not because they induce an actual improvement of the underlying Crohn's disease. An alternative theory is that antibiotics work in an anti-inflammatory/immune-modulating capacity.

Antibiotics are frequently used as primary therapy in the setting of perianal abscesses and fistulas (see Questions 40 and 41), as well as for **pouchitis** (inflammation of the ileal pouch after surgery for ulcerative colitis; see Question 51).

Pouchitis

inflammation of the ileal pouch.

Antibiotics are also used to treat bacterial overgrowth, which is a condition in which there is an overgrowth of normal bowel flora. Bacterial overgrowth occurs mostly in the setting of **intestinal stasis** caused by a stricture that disrupts the normal flow of intestinal contents through the intestine to the colon. Much like a still lake with an overgrowth of algae, intestinal stasis promotes the overgrowth of bacteria. Individuals with bacterial overgrowth develop diarrhea, cramps, bloating, and flatulence—similar symptoms to an IBD flare. Although bacterial overgrowth can be diagnosed by using a **hydrogen breath test**, most physicians make the diagnosis based upon the clinical presentation and use **empiric therapy**, treating with antibiotics.

Hydrogen breath test

a test to diagnose bacterial overgrowth.

Antibiotics are also used in patients with active Crohn's disease of the colon, but most often in addition to an aminosalicylate and not as primary therapy. Antibiotics are least often used for small bowel Crohn's disease. However, some physicians prescribe antibiotics as primary therapy for Crohn's disease regardless of the site of involvement.

Metronidazole (Flagyl) is one of the most commonly used antibiotics in Crohn's disease. It is usually dosed at 250 to 500 milligrams three to four times a day. Metronidazole's usefulness is limited by its side effects. Nausea, loss of appetite, and a metallic taste in the mouth are commonly experienced. These resolve when the dose is decreased or the drug is withdrawn. Long-term use of metronidazole can damage the nerves leading to the hands and feet, resulting in numbness and a tingling sensation. Although these effects usually are reversed when the drug is stopped, some individuals suffer permanent damage. For this reason, if you take metronidazole and develop symptoms of nerve damage, you should immediately stop the drug and inform your physician. The neurological effects of metronidazole are cumulative, so any person experiencing such symptoms should be considered allergic and should not take metronidazole again in the future. Alcohol should be strictly avoided by anyone on metronidazole; the combination of alcohol and metronidazole can cause you to get severely sick to the stomach.

Ciprofloxacin (Cipro) is a quinolone antibiotic and often is used in place of or along with metronidazole. It is usually dosed at 250 to 500 milligrams twice a day. Levofloxacin (Levaquin) is another quinolone antibiotic and is dosed at 250 to 500 milligrams once a day. Ciprofloxacin and levofloxacin are nearly as effective and usually much better tolerated because of their more favorable side effect profile; nausea, diarrhea, headache, and sensitivity to sunlight have been reported. Other antibiotics, such as rifaximin (Xifaxin), have also shown promise in the treatment of Crohn's disease.

25. Does having Crohn's disease or ulcerative colitis mean I will be on medication for my entire life?

Crohn's disease and ulcerative colitis are chronic, lifelong medical conditions and usually require long-term therapy. Although not every patient must be on medication all of the time, the majority of patients need some form of therapy most of the time. This is more so in patients with ulcerative colitis for which strong evidence supports that daily maintenance therapy significantly reduces the risk of a flare. Patients with ulcerative colitis who are in remission on sulfasalazine (Azulfidine), an aminosalicylate, azathioprine (Imuran) or 6-mercaptopurine (6-MP) have an 80–90% chance of remaining in remission, whereas those who stop taking medication have an 80–90% chance of having an **exacerbation** within a year. In addition, some scientific evidence supports the idea that daily maintenance therapy may reduce the risk of colon cancer.

Crohn's disease and ulcerative colitis are chronic, life-long medical conditions and usually require long-term therapy.

Although the scientific evidence supporting daily therapy with sulfasalazine or one of the newer aminosalicylates in Crohn's disease is not as strong as it is in ulcerative colitis, many physicians still prefer that their patients stay on maintenance therapy given that the risks of the drugs are small and that they may provide some protective benefit. Stronger evidence supports the role of daily maintenance therapy with azathioprine or 6-MP, although there are more potential side effects. The benefits of each drug must be carefully weighed against the risks for each individual patient. After surgery for Crohn's disease, in certain cases physicians may recommend medication to help delay or possibly prevent Crohn's disease from recurring.

Unfortunately, more hope than evidence supports this type of **prophylactic therapy**.

For patients with Crohn's disease and ulcerative colitis who take infliximab, strong evidence that supports using this drug both acutely to treat active symptoms and then chronically to maintain remission.

Other drugs such as prednisone and budesonide are useful in treating an acute flare but have a limited role in maintenance therapy because of eventual loss of effectiveness over time as well as the potential for long-term complications from chronic use, such as osteoporosis, hypertension, cataracts, and diabetes.

Ken's comment:

I've become accustomed to my daily medicine routine! I've been on a combination of sulfasalizine and azathioprine (Imuran) for several years now, and for me that seems to be the "magic formula" that has kept my ulcerative colitis in remission for several years. For me, remembering to take medicine a few times a day is way better than having to deal with a disease flare-up. And, I'm fully prepared to accept changes to my medications if my doctor so advises; again, having to adjust to a new medicine sure beats dealing with ulcerative colitis symptoms!

Also, the treatment options for IBD seem to be growing by the day. I've read of several new treatments that have been developed over the years, giving patients more and more ways to treat their symptoms. It's important as a patient to know what those options are and to discuss with your doctor which treatments are and aren't working. Also, make sure you know what medications you are on and know what side effects—if any—are associated with each treatment.

Jennifer's comment:

While living with Crohn's disease over the past decade and a half, I have been on and off a wide range of medications and have undergone two bowel resections [see Question 47]. During this time, I have learned (perhaps the hard way) that daily medications are a small inconvenience for maintaining a symptom-free existence.

After my second surgery, my gastroenterologist in New York prescribed a combination of Mesalamine (Asacol) and 6-MP in an effort to delay (and hopefully prevent) my Crohn's disease from recurring. I had only 4 symptom-free years between my first and second surgeries. Since beginning a daily regimen of Mesalamine and 6-MP more than 6 years ago, I have maintained my remission—that is, I have been symptom free and in exceptionally good health since my second surgery. This is all the evidence I need to continue taking medications for the rest of my life, if necessary. To me, this is a small price to pay for the chance to avoid the pain and discomfort of an active Crohn's flare-up.

26. I've heard that if you have IBD you can't take ibuprofen or naproxen. Is this true, and if it is, what can I do about my arthritis?

Ibuprofen and naproxen (Naprosyn) are part of a class of drugs called nonsteroidal anti-inflammatory drugs, or **NSAIDs**. NSAIDs are sold over the counter and are among the most commonly prescribed drugs in the world. They are frequently used for headaches, muscle aches, menstrual cramps, and joint pain and stiffness.

NSAID

nonsteroidal anti-inflammatory drug; anti-inflammatory medication commonly used to treat headaches and joint and muscle aches.

60

It is well known that NSAIDs can irritate the stomach and may lead to the development of **gastritis** and ulcers. In addition to stomach and duodenal ulcers, NSAIDs can also cause ulcers to form throughout the small bowel and colon, a condition called **NSAID enterocolopathy**. These ulcers are often confused with Crohn's disease because Crohn's disease also manifests as ulcers in the gastrointestinal tract.

NSAIDs have been reported to trigger IBD flares. For this reason, physicians often advise patients to avoid these types of drugs. Certainly, NSAIDs should be avoided if you have active IBD. However, for someone in remission, an occasional dose of ibuprofen or naproxen is unlikely to cause a Crohn's disease or ulcerative colitis flare. Some patients in remission do take NSAIDs on a chronic basis, such as for the treatment of chronic back pain, and do not suffer any ill effects. These individuals should be vigilant in monitoring for any signs of their Crohn's disease or ulcerative colitis becoming active.

NSAIDs have been reported to trigger IBD flares.

If you have Crohn's disease or ulcerative colitis, the best advice is to try to avoid NSAIDs even if you are in remission. If you do need anti-inflammatory medication, speak with your physician about an alternative therapy.

For those with IBD who also have joint pain, some of the medications used to treat Crohn's disease and ulcerative colitis, such as sulfasalazine and infliximab, are also helpful in arthritis. Finally, joint pains are commonly seen in Crohn's disease and ulcerative colitis and often improve with treatment directed at the underlying IBD.

27. Is it okay to use antidiarrheal drugs such as dephenoxylate/atropine (Lomotil) or loperamide (Imodium), and what other drugs are available to treat the symptoms of IBD?

Diarrhea is one of the most troubling and embarrassing symptoms of IBD. The urgent need to move one's bowels, always having to know where the bathroom is, and, at times, fecal **incontinence** can be both distressing and debilitating. Even just the fear of having diarrhea can make you housebound and greatly diminish your quality of life. For this reason, gaining control over your bowel function is one of the main goals in treating IBD. The first line of therapy is the anti-inflammatory and immune-modulating drugs discussed earlier. By treating the underlying IBD, the diarrhea should diminish and very often will resolve. In fact, better control of bowel function is actually one of the markers used to assess therapeutic effectiveness.

Antimotility drugs (see Table 6) such as loperamide (Imodium) and dephenoxylate/atropine (Lomotil) are invaluable tools in IBD therapy. For diarrhea that is more difficult to control, codeine and distilled tincture of opium (DTO) can also be used. These drugs are usually used in addition to anti-inflammatory and immune-modulating therapy. However, they may be used alone in the setting of isolated diarrhea with no other signs of active IBD, such as rectal bleeding, abdominal pain, weight loss, or anemia. Severely ill patients should avoid antimotility agents because their use could potentially precipitate toxic dilatation of the colon, a condition known as **toxic megacolon** (see

Incontinence

leakage of stool (fecal incontinence) or urine (urinary incontinence) as a result of a loss of control.

Gaining control over your bowel function is one of the main goals in treating IBD.

Antimotility drugs

class of drugs that slow down gastrointestinal motility; used to treat diarrhea.

Toxic megacolon

acute distention with air of the colon that usually occurs in the setting of severe colitis; can occur in Crohn's colitis, ulcerative colitis, or infectious colitis.

Table 6   Commonly Used Antidiarrheal Drugs and Their Usual Doses

Drug	Dose
loperamide HCL (Imodium)	1–2 tablets up to four times daily
diphenoxylate/atropine2.5 (Lomotil)	1–2 tablets up to four times daily
Codeine	30 mg, 1–2 tablets up to four times daily
DTO	5–15 drops up to four times daily

DTO, distilled tincture of opium.

Question 37). The main side effects of these drugs are constipation, dizziness, lightheadedness, and **somnolence**.

Cholestyramine (Questran) is an antidiarrheal agent that has been found to be especially helpful for patients with Crohn's disease after surgical **resection** of the ileum. The ileum is the last part of the small intestine just before the colon, and it is where **bile acids** and vitamin B_{12} are absorbed. Because the ileum is affected in 70% of patients with Crohn's disease, often part or all of it is removed when surgery becomes necessary (see Question 46). Removal of the ileum can result in malabsorption of both bile acids and vitamin B_{12}. Loss of vitamin B_{12} is easily treated by administration of B_{12} shots once a month or by placing B_{12} gel (Nascobal) in the nostrils once a week. The unabsorbed bile acids, however, reach the colon where they act as an irritant and cause the colon to produce increased amounts of fluid. As a result, you might begin to experience urgent and watery diarrhea, especially after meals. Cholestyramine functions by binding bile acids before they reach the colon, thus

Resection

the surgical removal of a segment of intestine.

Bile acids

digestive enzymes synthesized in the liver and absorbed in the ileum; individuals with ileal disease or ileal resection are unable to absorb bile acids, which then enter the colon where they act as an irritant that causes diarrhea.

Medications

63

preventing the colon from producing more fluid. Cholestyramine is dosed as a single packet or scoop (approximately 4 grams) and is best taken immediately before breakfast, but may also be taken before lunch and dinner as well. Its main side effect is constipation. Cholestyramine can also bind up any other medication that you might be taking, so take other drugs either one hour before or one hour after taking cholestyramine.

Fiber supplements, such as Metamucil, Citrucel, Konsyl, Benefiber, and Fiber Con, may be useful as well. Although you might usually think of using them primarily for constipation, they also function as bulking agents and may help by thickening up watery stool.

In addition to diarrhea, painful bowel spasms can also be very distressing. Effective therapy for the underlying IBD is usually sufficient to provide relief. **Antispasmodic drugs** such as dicyclomine (Bentyl) and hycosamine (Levsin) may also be helpful. As with the antidiarrheal drugs, antispasmodic drugs should not be used in severely ill patients. Individuals taking these drugs may experience dry mouth, dry eyes, and urinary retention as the predominant side effects.

Antispasmodic drugs

class of drugs used to relieve painful bowel spasm.

28. I've heard a lot lately about probiotics. Can these help patients with IBD?

Approximately 400 different types of bacteria naturally live in the digestive tract.

Approximately 400 different types of bacteria naturally live in the digestive tract. The colon contains more bacteria than the small bowel does, and the types of bacteria are different. Why do you have bacteria in your digestive tract? Overall, these "healthy" bacteria may be present to help to fight the unhealthy bacteria that occasionally attempt to invade the bowels. Some have theorized that these beneficial bacteria produce organic compounds that help to boost the immune system, fight inflammation, and inhibit the growth of harmful bacteria. One example of unhealthy bacteria is called **Clostridium difficile**, or **C. diff.** for short. If a person takes antibiotics for an unrelated reason, such as a respiratory infection, the antibiotics can alter the normal bacterial environment in the colon by indiscriminately wiping out both the good and bad bacteria. Unhealthy bacteria such as *C. diff.* then have the opportunity to gain a foothold, overpopulate the colon, and cause an infection. Symptoms from *C. diff.* can include crampy abdominal pain, excess gas, and explosive, foul-smelling frequent diarrhea. Usually the antibiotics metronidazole or vancomycin are used to treat a *C. diff.* infection.

Clostridium difficile (C. diff.) an unhealthy bacterium that can overpopulate the colon, usually as a result of antibiotic use, which leads to colitis symptoms that include diarrhea and cramps. It is treated by the antibiotics metronidazole or vancomycin.

The term *probiotic* means "for life" (as opposed to *anti*biotics). Although we have yet to identify the exact mechanism of **probiotics**, the idea is that ingesting live, healthy bacteria can help to repopulate the digestive tract and restore balance. Several different strains of bacteria are used in probiotic supplements, including *Lactobacillus acidophilus, Lactobacillus casei, Bifidobacterium*, and *Saccharomyces boulardii.* Yogurt contains lactobacillus and has often been used as a way to supply healthy bacteria to the digestive tract. However, the commonly available pasteurized versions generally are not adequate because most of the bacteria have been eliminated in the pasteurization process. Yogurts labeled as containing live cultures are probably closer to the probiotic supplements commercially available over the counter. Remember that if you are lactose intolerant,

*Although we have yet to identify the exact mechanism of **probiotics**, the idea is that ingesting live, healthy bacteria can help to repopulate the digestive tract and restore balance.*

you may want to avoid eating too much yogurt because it is a dairy product and contains lactose as well.

Probiotics have been used to treat various illnesses, including irritable bowel syndrome, travelers' diarrhea, *C. diff.* infection, and antibiotic-associated diarrhea. Even acne and vaginal yeast infections have reportedly improved with probiotic use. Probiotics are also being used in Crohn's disease and ulcerative colitis, particularly for those who have persistent diarrhea despite treatment and those who have small bowel bacterial overgrowth, a condition that occurs when bacteria overpopulate the small bowel and cause symptoms of bloating, gas, abdominal cramps, and loose stools. Although not much scientific evidence tells whether and how well probiotics work, they are not harmful and there is no downside to trying them.

Probiotics are taken as a daily supplement, usually two pills in the morning and two at night. They can be used for a short amount of time, such as before and during travel to avoid diarrhea, or can be taken indefinitely to combat illnesses, such as irritable bowel syndrome. Probiotics should not replace other medications that you may be taking for Crohn's disease and ulcerative colitis, but rather can act as a potentially helpful addition to your regimen. As with any over-the-counter natural supplement, probiotics are not regulated, which means quality, ingredients, and appropriate doses of each brand are not guaranteed. Often, when you walk into a pharmacy or health food store, you are bombarded with different types of probiotics, each one more expensive than the next. When in doubt, ask your doctor whether he or she feels probiotics would be helpful, and, if so, which types of probiotics he or she recommends.

PART FOUR

Cancer and Dysplasia

Am I more likely to get colon cancer if
I have ulcerative colitis?

Does Crohn's disease also increase my
risk for cancer?

What is dysplasia and how is it related to cancer?

More ...

29. Am I more likely to get colon cancer if I have ulcerative colitis?

If you have ulcerative colitis, you may be at an increased risk for developing colon cancer as compared to the general population. The degree of risk is determined by how long you have had ulcerative colitis and how much of the colon is involved (see Table 7). The greater amount of time you have had ulcerative colitis and the greater the extent of colonic involvement, the greater the likelihood that colon cancer will develop. An additional possible **risk factor** is **primary sclerosing cholangitis,** which is a liver disorder that is associated with Crohn's disease and ulcerative colitis. Interestingly, activity of disease is not considered to be a risk factor. In other words, having severe colitis does not make you more likely to develop colon cancer, and being in remission does not make you less likely. It should also be clearly stated that although individuals with ulcerative colitis are considered to be at increased risk, this is as compared to the general population in which the chance of getting colon cancer in a person's lifetime is approximately 1 in 20. Although having ulcerative colitis does place you at increased risk as compared to someone who does not have ulcerative colitis, the majority of ulcerative colitis patients still will not develop colon cancer.

If you have ulcerative colitis, you may be at an increased risk for developing colon cancer as compared to the general population.

Table 7   Risk Factors for Cancer in Patients with IBD

Duration of disease
Extent of disease
Primary sclerosing cholangitis
Activity of disease is *not* a risk factor

A direct relationship exists between the amount of time you have had ulcerative colitis and the likelihood that cancer will develop. Colon cancer complicating ulcerative colitis rarely occurs before a duration of illness of eight years. If your ulcerative colitis is limited to the left colon (left-sided colitis), risk of colon cancer occurring usually is not before 10 to 15 years duration of disease. What is not as clear is how high the risk actually is. Early studies found that the risk of colon cancer after 20 years of disease was 15% and after 30 years about 25%. More recent studies, however, show the risk at 20 years to be closer to 8%, and the risk at 30 years around 18%.

Another risk factor is the extent of colonic involvement. When ulcerative colitis is limited to the rectum, there does not seem to be an increased risk of cancer. The risk increases the farther up the inflammation extends into the colon and is highest when the entire colon is involved.

30. Does Crohn's disease also increase my risk for cancer?

As with ulcerative colitis, individuals with Crohn's disease that primarily affects the colon are also considered to be at higher risk for colon cancer than the general population. The risk factors are the same—duration of disease, extent of disease, and, possibly, primary sclerosing cholangitis. The probability of developing colon cancer is the same for Crohn's disease as it is for ulcerative colitis, assuming an equal amount of colon is involved for the same length of time. However, because in Crohn's disease less of the colon is usually

As with ulcerative colitis, individuals with Crohn's disease that primarily affects the colon are also considered to be at higher risk for colon cancer than the general population.

Cancer and Dysplasia

involved than in ulcerative colitis, the overall likelihood that a Crohn's disease patient will develop colon cancer is less than that of an ulcerative colitis patient.

Individuals with Crohn's disease may experience an increased incidence of lymphoma and small bowel cancer. However, because these are rarely found, it is difficult to determine how frequently lymphoma and small bowel cancer actually occur.

31. What is dysplasia and how is it related to cancer?

Dysplasia is a Greek word meaning "disordered formation or structure." It is a premalignant change that can be found on biopsy prior to the development of cancer in both Crohn's disease and ulcerative colitis. In dysplasia, cells lose their normal appearance and start to take on malignant characteristics. In almost all cases, the dysplastic cells eventually progress to become cancerous cells.

Dysplasia cannot be seen with the naked eye. It is a cellular change and, therefore, can be seen only under a microscope. This is why a biopsy is needed for diagnosis. Dysplasia is classified as low-grade, high-grade, and indeterminate (probably negative or probably positive) (see Table 8). Low-grade is the first stage of dys-

Table 8 Dysplasia Classification

High grade
Low grade
Indeterminate
• probably positive
• probably negative

plasia in which the cells appear more normal than malignant. High-grade is the second stage, and the cells are closer to being malignant. Indeterminate means that the pathologist interpreting the biopsy cannot determine whether dysplasia is present, often because of background inflammation, which is commonly seen in IBD and which obscures the picture. However, the pathologist often has a sense if the biopsy is more likely to be normal or more likely to be dysplastic, hence the qualifying statement—probably negative, or probably positive.

Although dysplasia can be seen only with the aid of a microscope, on occasion an abnormal area of the colon, such as a lesion or mass, can be visualized and biopsied. If dysplasia is found, this entity is known as a **DALM**—dysplasia-associated lesion or mass. In the setting of a DALM, even if the biopsy is interpreted as having only low-grade dysplasia, there is greater than a 50% chance that cancer is actually present. Therefore, given the high likelihood of cancer being found, all patients with a DALM should undergo a colectomy.

It is critical to understand that normal biopsies without dysplastic cells are not a guarantee that dysplasia or cancer is not present in the colon. Because dysplasia is invisible to the naked eye, usually no visibly abnormal area can be targeted, and therefore, the biopsies are taken randomly throughout the colon. As a result, there is a chance that dysplastic areas of the colon will be missed and that only normal areas are biopsied. This is known as a sampling error.

So what do you do if you have dysplasia? As previously stated, in the case of a DALM, colectomy is the standard recommendation. For high-grade dysplasia, colectomy is usually recommended as well. What to do in case of low-grade dysplasia is not as clear-cut. Because of sampling error and because some studies have shown that patients can progress from low-grade dysplasia straight to cancer without experiencing the high-grade dysplasia phase, many physicians suggest that all patients with low-grade dysplasia undergo a colectomy. Others believe that a single biopsy that shows low-grade dysplasia when all other biopsies are normal is not a strong enough reason to recommend removal of the colon. Coloring the picture is the over-all clinical setting. Because the risk of cancer is directly related to the duration and extent of disease, if low-grade dysplasia is found in an individual who has had extensive ulcerative colitis for 30 years, colectomy would probably be warranted. On the other hand, if low-grade dysplasia is found in an individual with only left-sided ulcerative colitis of 8 years duration, a wait-and-see approach might be more reasonable. In the end, the decision to have a colectomy for dysplasia rests with you, and how much risk you are willing to accept. For those who cannot live with the chance that they might be harboring cancerous or precancerous cells, colectomy may be the best choice. And for those who understand there are no guarantees and are not as uncomfortable living with a degree of uncertainty, the best choice may be close observation.

Polyps *are small, usually* **benign** *growths in the colon and are found in approximately 20% of Americans.*

32. Is a polyp the same thing as dysplasia?

Polyps are small, usually **benign** growths in the colon and are found in approximately 20% of Americans. There are two general types of colon polyps—hyperplastic and adenomatous. Hyperplastic polyps are thought not to be a precursor to colon cancer and for this reason are not commonly believed to be clinically significant. Adenomatous polyps (also known as adenomas), on the other hand, are considered to be neoplastic or precancerous polyps, although most never actually grow into cancers. Because it is impossible to tell with the naked eye which polyp is hyperplastic versus which is an adenoma, and because no way exists to predict which polyp will become cancerous, physicians tend to remove all colon polyps found during colonoscopy. Additionally, in most cases, this is considered "curative" in that studies have shown that removing colon polyps leads to a reduction in the rate of colon cancer. Psuedopolyps are a type of inflammatory polyps often found in IBD and do not lead to cancer.

Because an adenoma is a neoplastic or precancerous polyp, it is, by definition, dysplasia. This begs the question: in the setting of ulcerative colitis, how do you distinguish an adenoma from a DALM (dysplasia-associated lesion of mass) (see Table 9)? Often it can be difficult, even for an expert, to distinguish between the two. If the polyp looks like a small, simple polyp, if there is no dysplasia surrounding the polyp or elsewhere in the colon, and if it is found in an older individual with short duration of disease and limited extent of ulcerative colitis, it probably is a polyp and can be treated by removal (known as a polypectomy). Alternatively, if the polyp appears large and atypical, if there is surrounding dysplasia or dysplasia elsewhere in the colon, and if it is found in a younger individual with long duration of disease and extensive colitis, more likely it

Table 9   Characteristics of DALM versus Adenoma

Dalm	Adenoma
Younger individual	Older individual
Long duration of disease	Short duration of disease
Extensive UC	Limited UC
Larger polyp with atypical appearance	Smaller polyp with typical appearance

DALM, dysplasia-associated lesion or mass; UC, ulcerative colitis.

represents true dysplasia and should be treated with colectomy.

33. How do you screen for dysplasia and colon cancer in IBD?

All patients with ulcerative colitis or colonic Crohn's disease should be enrolled in a surveillance program to screen for dysplasia and cancer. Dysplasia is the precursor to colon cancer in both ulcerative colitis and Crohn's disease. Because it can be diagnosed only by biopsy, patients need to undergo periodic colonoscopies to obtain the biopsies. For patients with extensive colitis, it is recommended that surveillance colonoscopy start after 8 years of disease, and for left-sided colitis, after 10 to 15 years of disease. Colonoscopy with multiple biopsies should be performed every other year until year 20, at which time colonoscopy should be performed annually thereafter. If dysplasia or an adenoma is found, surveillance should be done on a more frequent basis. Individuals with Crohn's disease of the colon are at the same risk and should follow these same recommendations.

Ken's comment:

To be sure, no one enjoys a colonoscopy. But, it's one of the unfortunate but necessary things about living with IBD. For me, a colonoscopy every other year is a small price to pay for peace of mind that I am not showing signs of dysplasia or cancer, or is a relief should a colonoscopy show signs of dysplasia so that my doctor can recommend early-stage treatment. Colonoscopies are so routine these days, they are really little more than an inconvenience. And the preparation for the colonoscopy—flushing your bowel the night before the procedure—is much worse than the procedure itself!

It's easy to put off procedures like this. But the consequences of doing so can be great.

34. Should patients with Crohn's disease be screened for small bowel cancer?

Individuals with small bowel Crohn's disease have an increased incidence of small bowel cancer and lymphoma. However, because small bowel **malignancy** is rare, and because technically we are unable to adequately examine and biopsy the small bowel, it is not currently recommended to screen for small bowel cancer complicating Crohn's disease. However, even though there is no recommendation to screen for small bowel cancer, which means to look for cancer in all patients with small bowel Crohn's disease even if they are stable, patients who develop warning signs—unexplained iron deficiency anemia, for example—should still be investigated for the possibility of a cancer.

Cancer and Dysplasia

35. Can I do anything to prevent getting colon cancer?

Some scientific evidence indicates that long-term medical therapy with aminosalicylates may reduce the likelihood of developing colon cancer in ulcerative colitis.

Some scientific evidence indicates that long-term medical therapy with aminosalicylates may reduce the likelihood of developing colon cancer in ulcerative colitis. It is thought that chronic suppression of inflammation may inhibit the transformation of normal cells into dysplastic cells. Although the available data regards only aminosalicylates and not other drugs used to treat ulcerative colitis, many physicians extend these findings to immune-modulating therapy as well. Also, some suggest that nutritional therapy with folic acid and calcium may be protective, but this is "softer" data and the results may simply be based on chance occurrence. Based on these findings, it is reasonable to recommend that all ulcerative colitis patients stay on chronic drug therapy to help prevent the development of colon cancer. It may also be advisable to take a daily multivitamin containing folic acid and calcium.

Ken's comment:

In addition to following my doctor's therapy regimen, for me, regular exercise and a balanced diet are important, not only for preventing colon cancer but for staying as healthy as possible. When I'm feeling good and not experiencing a flare-up, I make it a point to exercise regularly and eat well, especially when I'm able to eat cancer-fighting foods like fresh fruits and vegetables. I also take a multivitamin every day and drink plenty of juice and water. Although IBD can present problems to eating healthy and exercising regularly, I've found that whenever you're healthy enough to do so, maintaining an overall healthy lifestyle is very important.

PART FIVE

Complications

How do I know if my bowel is perforated?

I heard that people with Crohn's disease can get something called a fistula. Can you tell me what this is?

I have ulcerative colitis and often pass blood with my bowel movements. Is this something I should worry about?

More ...

36. I have a friend with Crohn's disease who was operated on for a bowel obstruction. Does this occur often in Crohn's disease?

Crohn's disease is characterized by chronic intestinal inflammation, which can cause scar tissue to form within the intestinal tract. Over time, this process of inflammation leading to scarring may cause a segment of the intestinal tract to become narrowed; this is called a stricture or **stenosis**. When acute inflammation develops on top of a stricture, the intestine can become swollen causing it to become completely blocked, which is called a bowel obstruction (Table 10). Another way for a bowel obstruction to develop is if a patient with an intestinal stricture eats something that is difficult to fully digest, such as raw vegetables. This could potentially plug up the stricture and lead to an obstruction. Nuts, berries, popcorn, and unripe fruit are also known to do this.

Strictures in the small bowel are best seen with an upper GI small bowel series or with an enteroclysis,

When acute inflammation develops on top of a stricture, the intestine can become completely blocked, which is called a bowel obstruction.

Table 10   Major Complications Associated with Crohn's Disease and Ulcerative Colitis

Obstruction
Perforation
Hemorrhage
Sepsis
Fistula
Abscess
Toxic megacolon

which is an advanced type of small bowel series. Strictures in the colon can be diagnosed with either a barium enema or colonoscopy; virtual colonoscopy, which is a CT scan of the colon, may also show a stricture. A bowel obstruction is usually easily visualized on a simple abdominal X ray; CT scan of the abdomen can also be used and often provides additional information, such as the cause of the obstruction.

When a bowel obstruction occurs, patients usually experience intense abdominal pain, abdominal distention, little or no passage of stool or gas, and sometimes vomiting. Individuals in this scenario are almost always hospitalized both for treatment of the obstruction, as well as for monitoring for complications, such as an intestinal perforation (see Question 38). Treatment consists mostly of eating or drinking nothing so as not to worsen the obstruction, intravenous fluids for hydration, and intestinal decompression with nasogastric suction (a small, **nasogastric tube** is passed through the nose into the stomach and then is connected to a suctioning device). Intravenous corticosteroids are sometimes given as well. The majority of patients respond to this therapy.

When a bowel obstruction occurs, patients usually experience intense abdominal pain, abdominal distention, little or no passage of stool or gas, and sometimes vomiting.

Those who do not respond to therapy usually require surgery to relieve the obstruction. This type of surgery frequently involves resecting the segment of bowel that is obstructed. In another type of operation, rather than resect the stricture, the surgeon opens up or widens the stricture, which is called a **stricture-plasty**. This latter type of operation, however, is usually not performed in the setting of an emergency operation in a patient with a bowel obstruction. Strictureplasty is mostly done as an elective operation in a patient who may have multiple structures and for whom the surgeon wants to limit the amount of bowel removed.

A bowel obstruction can also develop as a result of an **adhesion**. An adhesion is the presence of scar tissue that has formed inside the **abdominal cavity** but outside of the intestines themselves. Adhesions are mostly seen after a prior abdominal operation of any type, such as appendectomy or hysterectomy, and are not peculiar to just Crohn's disease or ulcerative colitis. The treatment of a bowel obstruction from an adhesion is similar to that of an intestinal stricture: eating and drinking nothing, intravenous hydration, and nasogastric suction. Intravenous corticosteroids would be of little benefit in this setting.

When a patient with active Crohn's disease who also has had a prior abdominal operation presents with a bowel obstruction, it is often difficult to tell whether it is from an intestinal stricture or an adhesion. Fortunately, the treatment is similar for both problems and the majority of patients heal without the need for surgery.

37. What is toxic megacolon?

Toxic mega-colon is one of the most seri-ous but fortu-nately rare complications of IBD.

Toxic megacolon is one of the most serious but fortunately rare complications of IBD. More often seen in ulcerative colitis than in Crohn's disease, toxic megacolon is characterized by marked distention of the colon with air and is usually seen in an individual very ill from severe colitis. In addition to IBD, toxic megacolon can also be seen with infectious colitis.

Toxic megacolon may present spontaneously without any obvious precipitating factor. More often, however, it is caused by overuse of certain drugs that should not be used or that should be used sparingly in individuals with severe colitis. Examples include narcotics, such as morphine and oxycodone/acetaminophen (Percocet); antidiarrheals, such as loperamide HCL (Imodium) and diphenoxylate/atropine2.5 (Lomotil); antispasmodic drugs, such as dicyclomine HCL (Bentyl) and hyoscyamine sulfate (Levsin); and tricyclic antidepressant drugs, such as amitriptyline HCL (Elavil). Laxatives, especially the ones used as bowel prep prior to colonoscopy, should be strictly avoided. In the setting of severe colitis, colonoscopy in and of itself may also precipitate toxic megacolon; it should be performed only if the potential benefit is believed to justify the risk.

Patients with toxic megacolon appear ill and have severe abdominal pain and tenderness, distention, fever, rapid heart rate, low blood pressure, and an elevated white blood count. Abdominal X rays show the colon to be markedly distended with air.

Toxic megacolon is potentially life-threatening and needs to be treated aggressively to prevent even more ominous complications—**sepsis** (infection spreading through the bloodstream), colonic perforation with **peritonitis**, and/or shock. Patients need nasogastric suction to remove air from the bowel, IV fluids to prevent dehydration, and antibiotics to treat any infectious process. Also, IV corticosteroids are often used, especially in patients who have been taking oral corticosteroids prior to presentation. Immune-suppressing agents are usually avoided because of the possibility of concurrent infection. Patients who do not respond to therapy will need an urgent colectomy and **ileostomy**.

38. How do I know if my bowel is perforated?

Perforation (rupture of the bowel) is a rare complication of Crohn's disease and ulcerative colitis. Similar to toxic megacolon, it presents with the abrupt onset of abdominal pain, tenderness, and distention, fever, rapid heart rate, low blood pressure, and an elevated white blood count. Abdominal X rays show that air has escaped from the bowel through the perforation and has entered the abdominal cavity.

Patients presenting with a perforated bowel almost always undergo emergency surgery to identify the site of perforation, close the hole, or resect the diseased segment of bowel. In the case of an individual with Crohn's disease of the ileum that has perforated, an ileocolic resection (removal of the ileum, ileocecal valve, and part of the right colon) with reconnection of the remaining small bowel to the ascending colon is usually performed. A temporary ileostomy, however, may need to be created if the abdominal cavity is soiled or infected. For an ulcerative colitis patient who develops a perforation, a total colectomy with ileostomy is usually required.

39. What is sepsis, and why does it happen?

Sepsis is a serious medical condition that occurs when an overwhelming infection has spread through the bloodstream. In IBD, the infection usually originates in the gastrointestinal tract because that is the organ most affected by disease. Intestinal ulcers, the hallmark of Crohn's disease and ulcerative colitis, can burrow deep into the intestinal wall, which allows bacteria to seep out of the intestines and into the bloodstream. From there, the bacteria are disseminated throughout the body.

The signs and symptoms of sepsis include fever, chills, rapid heart rate, low blood pressure, and, at times, nausea, vomiting, and confusion. Septic shock occurs when the infection has caused the blood pressure to remain persistently low and adversely affects multiple organs such as kidneys, the liver, and lungs.

Antibiotics are administered to treat sepsis, and support for the failing organs is provided—dialysis in case of kidney failure, for example—until the body can support itself.

Jennifer's comment:

My experience with sepsis was one of the scariest side effects associated with my Crohn's disease. While attempting to combat what turned out to be an aggressive recurrence of my disease, I began experiencing fevers ranging between 102 and 104 degrees. Then while out with a friend one day, I began shaking and could not stop. By the time I made it home, I had spiked an extremely high fever; my boyfriend (now my husband) put me in a bath of cold water and called my doctor.

I was immediately put on oral antibiotics to treat the sepsis I had developed. Unfortunately, the fevers persisted and I was hospitalized to treat the infection with stronger antibiotics that are administered intravenously. It took 5 days in the hospital on antibiotics before my fever broke. We soon discovered that this massive infection in my bloodstream was the result of a perforated bowel.

40. I heard that people with Crohn's disease can get something called a fistula. Can you tell me what this is?

A fistula is a small tunnel or channel that forms between two structures in the body that are normally not connected.

A fistula is a small tunnel or channel that forms between two structures in the body that are normally not connected. In Crohn's disease, the most common type of fistula is a perianal fistula. A perianal fistula is when a tunnel forms between the lower rectum and the skin surrounding the anus. In women, fistulas may also form between the rectum and vagina. This is called a rectovaginal fistula. Other types of fistulas include channels forming between two sections of the small bowel (enteroenteric fistula), between the small bowel and the colon (enterocolonic fistula), between two parts of the colon (colocolonic fistula), between the colon and the bladder (colovesicular fistula), and between the small bowel and skin (enterocutaneous fistula). The reason a fistula may form is because in Crohn's disease the inflammatory process often involves the full thickness of the bowel wall. The inflamed bowel may then adhere to a nearby structure, such as the rectum to the vagina. In such a case, a small tunnel or fistula may develop between the two adherent structures.

The type of fistula and degree of symptoms determines what treatment is most appropriate. Fistulas between intestinal segments are mostly asymptomatic and are usually not treated beyond standard therapy for Crohn's disease. Perianal fistulas, rectovaginal fistulas, and colovesicular fistulas, on the other hand, usually cause a wide range of symptoms. Small, mildly symptomatic fistulas are usually treated with antibiotics. Complex and debilitating fistulas may require more intensive drug therapy with immune-modulating agents. Also, surgical techniques are often employed in treating complex fistula disease. On rare occasion, a **colostomy** or ileostomy may be required to divert the fecal stream away from the fistulas to give the fistulas a better chance of healing.

Fistulas are almost never seen in ulcerative colitis.

Fistulas are almost never seen in ulcerative colitis.

41. What is an anal fissure?

An anal fissure is a small cut or tear that can be seen in the anal canal. Although small, because the anus is extremely sensitive, an anal fissure can be very painful. Typically, you might experience a burning pain during or after a bowel movement and often find a streak of blood coating the stool and on the toilet paper. Anal fissures are seen most often when an individual with constipation strains to have a bowel movement and passes a hard stool, which creates a superficial tear in the anal canal. Anal fissures can also be found in individuals who have diarrhea; the constant bowel activity and frequent wiping traumatizes the area. You can apply a cortisone/anesthetic cream as acute treatment of an anal fissure. In the long term, better regulating

Because the anus is extremely sensitive, an anal fissure can be very painful.

your underlying bowel pattern to avoid both constipation and diarrhea is best.

Anal fissures are more commonly seen in Crohn's disease than in ulcerative colitis. In the setting of Crohn's disease, an anal fissure may represent active Crohn's disease in the anus itself. As such, anal fissures complicating Crohn's disease are usually more resistant to treatment than an anal fissure in an individual who does not have Crohn's disease. The initial treatment for an anal fissure in an individual with Crohn's disease is similar to the treatment in someone without Crohn's disease, as described earlier. If the anal fissure does not respond, additional drug therapy with antibiotics and immune-modulating agents may be employed. Less commonly, anal surgery may be indicated.

42. I have Crohn's disease and often get abscesses around my rectum. What exactly is an abscess and how is it treated? Can I get abscesses in other places?

An abscess can form at any site in the body, but in Crohn's disease it is most often seen around the rectum and anus and is referred to by various names— anorectal abscess, perianal abscess, or perirectal abscess.

An abscess is a localized infection, or collection of pus, that your body has walled off, much like a pimple. An abscess can form at any site in the body, but in Crohn's disease it is most often seen around the rectum and anus and is referred to by various names—anorectal abscess, perianal abscess, or perirectal abscess. In an anorectal abscess, the infection arises in the tissue surrounding the anus and rectum. Patients often experience a throbbing and constant rectal pain that is exacerbated when sitting. They may also feel a lump around the anus. If the abscess spontaneously drains, a fistula may be formed. The most common sites of drainage are around the anus (perianal fistula), and in a woman, into the vagina (rectovaginal fistula). Fistulas can track under the skin to more distant sites, such as the scrotum in a man and the vulva in a woman. To prevent these more complex fistulas from forming, prompt surgical drainage should be performed. While a fistula to the skin might still develop at the site of the drainage, it is likely be less debilitating than a fistula to the vagina, vulva, or scrotum. Antibiotics are usually prescribed as well.

Some individuals can develop a deeper abscess around the rectum. In these patients, the abscess has a more insidious presentation with deep rectal or lower abdominal discomfort, back pain, and/or fever and absence of a palpable lump around the anus. This type of abscess can often be identified by rectal exam. Because a rectal exam in this situation may be extremely painful, not infrequently patients are taken to the operating room to have a rectal exam after being anesthetized, which is called an **EUA**, or **evaluation under anesthesia**. At the same time, the surgeon can also incise and drain the abscess without causing the patient any discomfort. In addition to draining the abscess, the surgeon may decide to place a wick or drain in the abscess to allow it to slowly heal from the inside out. Otherwise, the abscess might close superficially on the skin side without fully closing internally, thus allowing for the potential that the abscess will re-form. The surgeon may also choose to place a **seton**, a small, thin, flexible piece of plastic tubing that is inserted through the skin and into the abscess, out the abscess, into the rectum, and then out through the anus where the two ends are tied

Complications

together. This is usually performed in the case of a large or recurring abscess to allow for long-term drainage so as to prevent the abscess from re-forming. The seton can be left in place for weeks to months and can be easily removed in the office after the drainage has stopped.

Other modalities used to diagnose a deep abscess include CT scan, MRI, and endorectal ultrasound.

Sometimes a chronic abscess or fistula may develop. In these cases, the patient may be given chronic antibiotics, often for many months. In addition, other drugs including immune-modulating agents are usually prescribed for such patients.

43. I have really bad hemorrhoids and something my doctor calls a skin tag. Are these common in someone with IBD?

Hemorrhoids are actually clumps of engorged veins in the anal canal, much like the varicose veins that commonly appear in the legs of some people. Hemorrhoids can also be seen in individuals with both chronic diarrhea and constipation. They are believed to be formed as a result of high pressure in the lower rectum and anus, which results when a person with diarrhea or constipation constantly bears down to have a bowel movement. Also, hemorrhoids are frequently seen in women after pregnancy as a result of their bearing down to deliver, as well as in fighter pilots who bear down to counteract high G (gravitational) forces during flight. Because IBD patients often have diarrhea, hemorrhoids are not uncommon. When hemorrhoids become engorged with blood, they can bleed. When blood clots within the hemorrhoids, the hemorrhoids are said to be thrombosed, which can be a very painful condition. The best therapy is to treat the underlying diarrhea or constipation. Topical therapy with **steroid** and anesthetic creams is often helpful as well.

Skin tags are single or multiple tags of excess anal or perianal tissue. They can develop after a **thrombosed hemorrhoid**, after anal operations, or they can form for no particular reason (i.e., they are idiopathic). As with hemorrhoids, treatment is aimed at improving the underlying bowel disorder. Local therapy with creams and ointments may also be used.

44. I go to the bathroom so much that I get a lot of itching and irritation. What can I do to treat this?

Perianal dermatitis, or irritation of the skin around the anus, is commonly found in individuals with chronic bowel problems. This is something that many patients have, yet few talk about. It can be caused by either dry skin from frequent wiping or moist skin from anal seepage. Also, standard bathroom soap, especially perfumed soap, may irritate this area as well. After having a bowel movement, individuals with perianal irritation should first use a moist wipe and then finish wiping with toilet paper. For someone who suffers from anal seepage, better control of bowel function to prevent seepage should be the initial therapy. Use of talcum powder can also help to dry out the area. Other helpful hints include practicing good general anal hygiene by showering with a hand shower, and applying A&D Ointment or Desitin at night. Topical corticosteroid creams and ointments for individuals with intense perianal dermatitis may be helpful in the short term. However, topical steroid treatment should not be used for more than

1 to 2 weeks—any longer, and **atrophy** (i.e., thinning) of the skin may ensue. Fungal infections can also develop in any moist, closed area, such as between the buttocks or under the breasts. For this reason, if the simple measures outlined here do not lead to improvement within a week or 2, seek professional medical attention to exclude a fungal infection.

Rectal bleeding is one of the cardinal symptoms of ulcerative colitis.

45. I have ulcerative colitis and often pass blood with my bowel movements. Is this something I should worry about?

Rectal bleeding is one of the cardinal symptoms of ulcerative colitis. Red blood coating or mixed with stool, bloody diarrhea, or passing red blood with clots is commonly found and indicates that colitis is more active. As you would expect, rectal bleeding often leads to a great deal of worry and concern; you might be wondering, "Am I going to bleed to death?" Fortunately, like a drop of red dye in a glass of water, passing blood per rectum usually looks much worse than it really is. Most ulcerative colitis patients with rectal bleeding have only mild anemia. More severe anemia can be seen in chronic ulcerative colitis that has not been adequately treated and in individuals with severe **hemorrhagic colitis** that requires them to be hospitalized. Symptoms of more significant bleeding that can result in severe anemia include lightheadedness, dizziness, and fatigue. Anemia can be confirmed with a blood test to check the hemoglobin or hematocrit level, which is part of a complete blood count (CBC).

Successful treatment of ulcerative colitis leads to resolution of both rectal bleeding and anemia. For individuals with more severe iron deficiency anemia, iron supplementation is often added. Unfortunately, iron pills can also cause gastrointestinal side effects, such as nausea, constipation, and black-colored stools. If you cannot tolerate iron pills, you may receive intravenous iron instead. Hospitalized patients with severe hemorrhagic colitis and profound anemia usually require blood transfusions along with aggressive medical therapy. Urgent colectomy may be needed if the medical therapy is unsuccessful.

Rectal bleeding is not seen as frequently with Crohn's disease as it is in ulcerative colitis. Anemia, on the other hand, is a common finding in Crohn's disease and is treated in a similar fashion. Severe bleeding complicating Crohn's disease is seen infrequently. As with ulcerative colitis, blood transfusions, aggressive medical therapy, and, potentially, surgery may be necessary.

Patients with ulcerative colitis or Crohn's disease can, at times, show signs of bleeding unrelated to their IBD. The passage of dark, tarry stool (medically called **melena**) suggests blood loss from the upper part of the gastrointestinal tract. This is most commonly from an ulcer, which can be seen in up to one in eight Americans. Bleeding from an ulcer is potentially life-threatening; anyone with this type of blood loss should report it immediately to his or her physician.

Bleeding from an ulcer is potentially life-threatening; anyone with this type of blood loss should report it immediately to his or her physician.

PART SIX

Surgery

What types of operations are performed
in Crohn's disease?

How often does Crohn's disease recur after surgery,
and is there any way to prevent it?

What types of operations are performed
in ulcerative colitis?

More . . .

46. What is the role of surgery in Crohn's disease?

Although Crohn's disease is usually adequately treated with medical therapy, approximately 70–80% of patients will still need to undergo surgery at some point in their lifetime. Surgery becomes necessary when medical treatment is no longer able to keep the symptoms of Crohn's disease under control, or when a complication arises.

Although Crohn's disease is usually adequately treated with medical therapy, approximately 70–80% of patients will still need to undergo surgery at some point in their lifetime.

When a person's Crohn's disease is no longer responsive to medical therapy, you, your gastroenterologist, and a surgeon should jointly make the decision whether to perform surgery. To achieve the best outcome, all three parties should be in agreement. Often, you may want surgery because you are frustrated by your illness and feel that you won't get better. However, your physicians may encourage you to be patient, knowing from experience and extensive training that the medicine might need more time to work fully. In addition, because Crohn's disease has such a high postoperative **recurrence** rate, physicians are often reluctant to recommend surgery until all reasonable medical options have been exhausted. At other times, however, a physician may recommend surgery knowing that there are no good medical options left, while you may not yet be ready psychologically for an operation.

One of the factors that physicians take into account when deciding on surgery is whether you are on any medication that either has caused or has the potential to cause you harm. Prednisone, for example, can cause a multitude of side effects, many of which can be very serious. For this reason, surgery is often considered for an individual who has become prednisone dependent to allow the patient to discontinue this drug and avoid any potentially deleterious effects.

When a complication occurs, the decision to have surgery is more clear-cut. When bowel perforation, bowel obstruction, toxic megacolon, sepsis, or an abscess develops, surgery is almost always indicated. This is not to say that nonoperative therapy might not be attempted, but that the threshold to operate is much lower and the decision is usually made much quicker.

Jennifer's comment:

The decision to undergo surgery the first time was actually a very easy one for me to make. After being diagnosed and living with Crohn's for just over a year, I knew my body was not responding to any of treatments that had been pre-scribed. The pain I was living with was getting worse instead of better despite the multitude of medications I had been on and the frequent hospitals stays spent hooked up to intravenous fluids intended to relieve the inflammation in my intestinal tract. I was 18 years old, preparing to leave for college, and miserable.

I'll never forget the day I asked Dr. Warner to consider sur-gery. We had discussed this option together in the past, but only as a last resort. On this day, I sat in his office with my mother desperate for relief from the constant pain I was in. I was not worried about the implications or side effects of surgery; rather, I was willing to try just about anything to rid my body of this disease. Dr. Warner (and my parents) had more serious reservations than me. Dr. Warner explained that this was not a decision to be made lightly, especially for a teenager—someone with many years ahead of her and with a finite amount of intestines to operate on if the need for surgery became necessary later on in life. That said, he agreed that it had seemed we had run out of medical options, and it was time to consider surgery. He then ordered a series of X rays that confirmed what we all feared to be the case—I was no longer responding to my medications and my disease was progressing.

Shortly thereafter I underwent my first major surgery—an ileocolic resection to remove the diseased portion of my intestine. Five years later, I underwent a second bowel resection as a result of an aggressive recurrence of my disease. Both surgeries provided me immediate relief of my disease, but the recovery process was difficult. In both instances, I was in the hospital for about 7 days, and then at home for another 5 weeks recuperating. The outcome, however, was well worth my time out of commission.

I have never been scared by the prospect of surgery, largely because I had complete faith in the doctors caring for me and the fact that I knew surgery offered me time without painful Crohn's symptoms. Although surgery was utilized as a last resort to treat my disease in both instances, I am grateful I had this option because it proved to be an effective longer-term therapy for me.

In Crohn's disease, the most common type of operation performed is to surgically remove the diseased segment of intestine, which is known as a bowel resection.

47. What types of operations are performed in Crohn's disease?

In Crohn's disease, the most common type of operation performed is to surgically remove the diseased segment of intestine, which is known as a bowel resection. The two healthy ends of intestine are then sewn or stapled together to form what is called an **anastomosis**, which is a surgical connection between the two structures. Sometimes, an anastomosis cannot be created; if this is the case, an ileostomy or colostomy may be required. An ileostomy is when the surgeon brings the small bowel (usually the ileum) through the abdominal wall and attaches it to the skin. The end of the ileum is made to protrude through the skin to form what is called a **stoma**. A colostomy is when the colon is used in place of the ileum. Waste products are then collected into an external pouch, or bag (see Figure 3). One of the main reasons that an ileostomy or colostomy is formed rather than an anastomosis is the presence of an intra-abdominal infection (i.e., infection within the abdominal cavity). If the anastomosis were to become infected, it could break down and leak bowel contents into the abdomen. This could cause peritonitis, an even more severe intra-

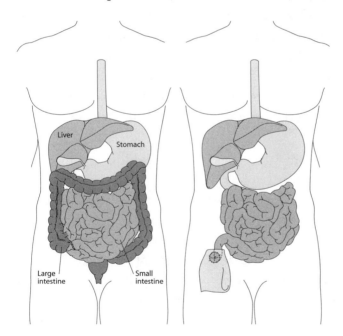

FIGURE 3 Normal anatomy (l) and anatomy after proctocolectomy and ileostomy (r).

abdominal infection. Therefore, rather than run this risk, the surgeon may choose to create an ileostomy or colostomy until the initial intra-abdominal infection has resolved. Then, at a later time, the surgeon will perform a second operation to take down the ileostomy or colostomy and form an anastomosis between the two remaining sections of bowel. At times, however, it may be necessary to have a permanent ileostomy or colostomy.

A colostomy is sometimes created in the setting of severe perianal Crohn's disease. When a patient becomes debilitated from recurrent perianal abscesses and fistulas that do not heal with maximal medical therapy, a colostomy may be formed to divert the fecal stream away from the rectum and anus. This improves the chances of the abscesses and fistulas to heal because the area is no longer bathed with stool. Unfortunately, once the colostomy is taken down and bowel continuity restored, the abscesses and fistulas often recur. For this reason, a diverting colostomy created to protect the perianal area is often permanent.

Strictureplasty is another operation commonly performed in Crohn's disease. In this operation, the surgeon widens or opens up a small bowel stricture to relieve the patient of obstructive symptoms. Strictureplasty is often referred to as bowel-preserving surgery because the diseased bowel is not removed. This allows patients to preserve more of their intestines. Usually, the surgeon decides to perform a resection versus a strictureplasty during the operation based upon the operative findings.

Intestinal **bypass** is an operation for Crohn's disease that is less commonly performed today. In this operation, rather than resect the diseased segment of intestine, the surgeon bypasses the bowel by connecting the healthy intestine above the diseased segment to the healthy intestine below. As an example, for ileal Crohn's disease, the surgeon would bypass the Crohn's disease by connecting the healthy intestine above the diseased ileum to the healthy colon below. Unfortunately, many patients developed cancer in the bypassed segment of intestine, which is why this operation is now almost never performed.

48. How often does Crohn's disease recur after surgery, and is there any way to prevent it?

One of the most frustrating aspects of Crohn's disease is that a patient can never be completely cured of it. After undergoing intestinal resection and creation of an anastomosis, the vast majority of patients develop a recurrence of their Crohn's disease. Interestingly, when an ileocolic resection (removal of the lower ileum and first part of the colon, the most common operation for Crohn's disease) is performed for Crohn's disease of the ileum, recurrence of Crohn's disease is almost always found above the anastomosis on the small bowel side; it is unusual for Crohn's disease to recur below or on the colon side of the anastomosis. On the other hand, when the resection is done in the setting of Crohn's disease involving the colon, the recurrence can be seen on either or both sides of the anastomosis. Also, Crohn's disease tends to follow patterns. If the patient had a short stricture in the ileum before surgery, the recurrence after surgery will probably be a

One of the most frustrating aspects of Crohn's disease is that a patient can never be completely cured of it.

short stricture as well. The reason that Crohn's disease behaves in such a predictable fashion after surgery has never been understood.

What is the rate of postoperative recurrence? After a resection, approximately 20% of patients develop symptoms of Crohn's disease at 2 years, 30% at 3 years, and 50% at 5 years. This is also called the clinical recurrence rate. The endoscopic recurrence rate is much higher. If a colonoscopy was performed on every patient after surgery, signs of a recurrence could be found in up to 70% in 1 year and 85% in 3 years. The frequency of recurrence after an ileostomy is much lower—about 10% to 20% at 10 years. However, once the ileostomy is reversed and an anastomosis is created, the recurrence rate increases.

After a resection, approximately 20% of patients develop symptoms of Crohn's disease at 2 years, 30% at 3 years, and 50% at 5 years.

Is there any way to prevent a recurrence? If we could make only one recommendation, it would be to stop smoking. Cigarette smoking significantly increases the risk of a recurrence; quitting smoking reduces this risk. In addition, there is some evidence to suggest that medical therapy with aminosalicylates or immune-modulating drugs could possibly reduce the likelihood of a recurrence. More scientific evidence is needed before this can be recommended with greater confidence. For now, the decision to recommend postoperative prophylactic drug therapy in hopes of preventing or delaying a recurrence must be made on an individual basis. In an individual who has had extensive or multiple intestinal resections, prophylactic therapy with an aminosalicylate or immune-modulating drug may be reasonable. On the other hand, in an individual who has had only a single, limited resection, postsurgical prophylactic therapy may offer only marginal benefit.

Jennifer's comment:

I felt so good in the years following my first surgery that the idea of a recurrence was unfathomable. But I was not lucky enough to beat the odds; I became a statistic. Approximately 5 years after my first bowel resection, symptoms of my disease returned.

By this time I was in my early twenties, living a relatively healthy lifestyle and focused on a new-found career track in New York City; I did not believe I had time to be sick. In fact, I did not believe I was sick at all. I actually convinced myself that the pains in my intestine were just the result of stress or a "bad day" rather than an indication of a recurrence.

The worst thing I have ever done to myself is ignore my Crohn's symptoms. By the time my boyfriend (now my husband) convinced me to talk to my doctor about my symptoms, it was too late. My disease was progressing at an aggressive rate, attacking my body, and not responding to medical treatment. By the time I was admitted to the hospital for surgery, I was septic and the disease had perforated my bowel, forming an infection in the lining of a muscle in my back. The day before my operation, at the ripe age of 24, the surgeon delivered the most devastating news of all—given the state of the infection raging through my body, there was a very good chance I would wake up with a colostomy.

I was incredibly fortunate. The doctors were able to remove the infection along with the diseased bowel without the aid of a temporary colostomy. However, I learned a very important lesson that year and have since accepted the harsh, unpredictable reality of this disease.

Today I know that I am not cured; I am in remission. Despite 6 healthy, pain-free years (and a hope that with daily medications I may be beating the odds this time), I know that my next recurrence may be only a few days or weeks away. Although I choose not to live my life focused on the "what-ifs," I now make sure to report any unusual pain or discomfort promptly to Dr. Warner. I am determined never to experience the type of nightmare I lived through in New York again.

49. What is the role of surgery in ulcerative colitis?

Although ulcerative colitis usually can be treated successfully with medical therapy, approximately 25–35% of individuals require surgery. As with Crohn's disease, surgery becomes necessary when medicines are no longer able to maintain adequate control of symptoms or when a complication occurs. However, unlike Crohn's disease, surgery for ulcerative colitis is considered curative because once the colon has been removed, the colitis does not recur.

Although ulcerative colitis usually can be treated successfully with medical therapy, approximately 25–35% of individuals require surgery.

More than 95% of surgery performed in ulcerative colitis is done so electively because of patients' chronic, unremitting symptoms that cannot be adequately treated with medicines. As such, the decision to operate is based on the individual's quality of life and not on rigid criteria. For some individuals, 8 to 10 loose bowel movements per day are severely restricting— they become housebound, cannot work, travel, go out with friends, or care for their children. For others, the same frequency of bowel movements is more inconvenient than disabling, and they are able to go about their daily activities with little or no restriction.

As with Crohn's disease, the type of medication the patient is taking is another factor in the decision whether to operate. Prednisone dependence is often a reason to go to surgery, both because of side effects the patient may experience and out of concern for potential long-term complications, such as osteoporosis, hypertension, cataracts, and diabetes. In addition, some patients with ulcerative colitis choose to have surgery simply to avoid having to take immune-modulating drugs, such as azathioprine (Imuran) or 6-mercaptopurine (6-MP). Still others prefer to exhaust all available medical options and consider surgery only as a last resort.

Less than 5% of surgery performed in ulcerative colitis is performed for a complication of the disease. Perforation, **hemorrhage**, sepsis, and toxic megacolon rarely occur; bowel obstruction is almost never seen. Dysplasia and cancer are infrequent complications of ulcerative colitis.

50. What types of operations are performed in ulcerative colitis?

Surgery for ulcerative colitis involves removal of the entire rectum and colon, which is called a **procto-colectomy**. One frequent question patients ask is why the entire rectum and colon needs to be removed and not simply perform a more limited resection of only the diseased segment as is done in Crohn's disease. A proctocolectomy is performed for two main reasons. First, because the rectum is always involved in ulcerative colitis, the rectum almost always needs to be removed along with the portion of inflamed colon. Then, the healthy colon must connect directly to the

*Surgery for ulcerative colitis involves removal of the entire rectum and colon, which is called a **procto-colectomy**.*

anus, a procedure known as a coloanal anastomosis. This procedure is technically difficult and leads to a very poor functional outcome. (This would also be true in the case of Crohn's disease involving the rectum if the rectum were removed.) Second, in ulcerative colitis after limited colonic resection, there is a very high recurrence rate, which almost always leads to removal of the remainder of the colon anyway. Conversely, an individual with Crohn's disease could go years before having a recurrence after a limited colonic resection.

Total proctocolectomy with ileostomy is a widely recommended and performed operation for ulcerative colitis. It is curative, and patients can lead a long, happy, and healthy life. Unfortunately, some patients have a psychological barrier to living with an ileostomy. When possible, patients faced with the need for this surgery should be offered the opportunity to meet with other individuals living with an ileostomy. It is vital that patients be given the needed support from their family, physicians, stomal therapist, and support groups to help cope with this change. In the end, while prior-to-surgery patients often may have felt trapped by their disease, after surgery most patients feel liberated because they are finally able to work, play, travel, spend time with their family, and lead a productive life.

As an alternative to having a permanent ileostomy, patients may be given the option of having a **restorative proctocolectomy** (see Figure 4) in which an internal pouch, or reservoir, is created from the small bowel and is attached to the anus (remember, the small bowel and anus are healthy and are not involved in ulcerative colitis). Also known as an **ileal pouch anal anastomo-**

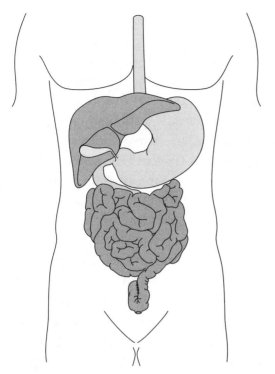

FIGURE 4 Ileal pouch-anal anastomosis. This is also called a "restorative" proctocolectomy.

sis, or the **J-pouch** (because it is shaped like the letter *J*), this operation enables the individual have bowel movements through the anus. This operation is usually performed in two stages. In the first stage, the colon and rectum are removed down to the anus. The ileum is then used to construct a pouch that is connected to the anus. A temporary ileostomy is created to allow the ileal pouch anal anastomosis to heal. Six to eight weeks later, the patient is brought back for the second stage of the operation when the temporary ileostomy is taken down and intestinal continuity is restored. Severely ill and malnourished patients undergo the operation in three stages—stage 1, removal of the colon with formation of an ileostomy; stage 2, **proctectomy**,

Ileal pouch anal anastomosis

operation performed mostly in ulcerative colitis in which part of the ileum is used to construct an internal pouch that is connected to the anus.

removal of the rectum, creation of an ileal pouch, and anastomosis of the pouch to the anus; and stage 3, taking down of the ileostomy. Some surgeons perform the operation in only one stage, but without a temporary ileostomy to divert the fecal stream away from the ileal pouch anal anastomosis, patients run a greater risk of breakdown of the anastomosis and subsequent pelvic sepsis. If pelvic sepsis occurs, the ileal pouch more than likely will not function optimally; eventually the pouch will need to be removed and the patient would then need a permanent ileostomy.

After surgery, patients have on average six to eight bowel movements per day of either a loose or putty-like consistency. It is common for patients to have to move their bowels one to two times each night, and some individuals have nocturnal seepage and have to wear a pad. To slow down the frequency of bowel movements and prevent dehydration, many individuals chronically take antidiarrheal medications, such as Imodium or Lomotil, and drink electrolyte-based fluids, such as Gatorade.

How do you decide which operation to have? This should be a joint decision between you, your gastroenterologist, and the surgeon. At times, technical factors make an ileal pouch anal anastomosis unlikely to be successful, in which case a total proctocolectomy with ileostomy would be the operation of choice. In the end, however, it often comes down to a trade-off between living with the inconveniences of an ileostomy versus the inconveniences of an ileal pouch.

51. What is pouchitis, and how is it treated?

Pouchitis is inflammation of the mucosa, or inside lining, of the ileal pouch and is the most common complication of pouch surgery. Eventually occurring in up to half of all pouch patients, pouchitis can be mild with just an increase in frequency of bowel movements, or as severe as a full-blown flare of ulcerative colitis with watery diarrhea, **urgency**, rectal bleeding, abdominal cramps, fever, weight loss, and **arthralgias** (joint pains). Other **extraintestinal manifestations** may be seen as well.

Patients who develop these symptoms should undergo an endoscopic examination of the pouch to confirm the diagnosis. Pouchitis appears as inflamed mucosa similar to that seen in ulcerative colitis. A biopsy may also be obtained during the endoscopic examination to help further characterize the inflammation. If the pouch appears normal on endoscopic examination, the physician should look for other potential causes for the patient's symptoms. Because an intestinal infection can mimic pouchitis, stool studies should always be obtained. Crohn's disease involving the small bowel above the pouch, irritable bowel syndrome, celiac sprue, and dietary indiscretion are just some of the other possibilities.

The cause of pouchitis is unknown, just as the causes of ulcerative colitis and Crohn's disease are unknown. Some believe that pouchitis is from an overgrowth of bacteria in the pouch, which may be why pouchitis often improves with antibiotics. Others feel that pouchitis

Surgery

Extraintestinal manifestations
signs of IBD that are found outside of the gastrointestinal tract.

represents a form of inflammatory bowel disease of the pouch. Interestingly, pouchitis is seen only after pouch surgery for IBD. It does not develop in patients who have had an ileal pouch anal anastomosis for **familial polyposis,** which is a disorder in which hundreds of pre-cancerous polyps form in the colon, necessitating **prophylactic colectomy** to prevent colon cancer from developing. The fact that pouchitis only develops in IBD patients suggests that it has an autoimmune origin.

How is pouchitis treated? Antibiotics are the most common treatment, with metronidazole and ciprofloxacin the most often used. Most patients respond after 1 or 2 weeks of therapy, although individuals with chronic or recurrent pouchitis may require long-term antibiotic therapy. Other antibiotics that have also been reported to be beneficial include clarithromycin (Biaxin), erythromycin, tetracycline, and amoxicillin (Augmentin). In addition to antibiotics, drugs used to treat ulcerative colitis have also been used to treat pouchitis with varying degrees of success. We have found topical therapy with hydrocortisone acetate combined with sulfasalazine to be particularly helpful. Corticosteroid and mesalamine (Rowasa) enemas, aminosalicylates, prednisone, budesonide, azathioprine, 6-mercaptopurine (6-MP), and infliximab may also be beneficial.

Not infrequently, some patients have the symptoms of pouchitis, but yet have a relatively normal-appearing pouch on endoscopy. In these cases, the patients may be experiencing spasm of the pouch, much in the way that someone with irritable bowel syndrome experiences abdominal discomfort and diarrhea (see Question 13). For this reason, drugs used to treat irritable bowel syndrome are often helpful in this setting: antispasmodic drugs, such as hyoscyamine sulfate and dicyclomine HCL; anticholinergic antidepressants, such as amitriptyline HCL; and antidiarrheal drugs, such as loperamide HCL and diphenoxylate/atropine 2.5.

Dietary indiscretion is another potential cause of pouchitis symptoms that occur with a normal-appearing pouch. Individuals with an ileal pouch have to be careful not to eat or drink substances that are known to cause diarrhea, such as caffeinated coffee and tea, and too much fresh fruit and raw vegetables. In some individuals, it is simply the quantity of fluid intake that is the culprit. The main function of the colon is fluid and electrolyte absorption. Individuals with an ileal pouch no longer have a colon and, there-fore, have less capacity to absorb fluid. For instance, one gentleman in his mid-50s was referred for severe diarrhea after ileal pouch surgery. On detailed questioning he was found to be drinking two 2-liter bottles of soda a day—given that he was asking his pouch to absorb 4 liters of soda each day, no wonder he was having severe diarrhea.

52. What are some of the other complications found after ileal pouch surgery?

Although many of the complications seen after ileal pouch surgery are those commonly found after any abdominal or pelvic operation, some are unique to the ileal pouch.

Bowel obstruction can occur after any abdominal operation as a result of the formation of adhesions, which are fibrotic bands of scar tissue that may develop within the abdominal cavity. A loop of intestine can twist around the fibrotic bands, leading to an obstruction. Unique to ileal pouch surgery, a bowel obstruction can also occur as a result of a kinking of the loop of ileum leading into the pouch itself. Whereas a bowel obstruction from adhesions usually resolves with nonoperative management, this unique type of obstruction often requires a surgical correction. Overall, small bowel obstruction can be seen in 20% of patients after ileal pouch surgery.

A stricture at the anastomosis between the ileal pouch and anus can also develop. Although a stricture may form at any anastomosis, they seem to occur more frequently at the pouch-anal anastomosis. A physician can easily treat this by dilating the stricture by using either a finger or an endoscopic balloon.

An abscess or fistula can be seen following pouch surgery, as well. This can be either a result of infection from an **anastomotic leak** or from Crohn's disease in the pouch. An anastomotic leak is when the anastomosis breaks down, usually because of an infection, and intestinal bacteria leak out, causing an even worse infection. It is often difficult to tell if the abscess or fistula is caused by an anastomotic leak or by Crohn's disease. If the abscess or fistula is from an anastomotic leak, it usually presents shortly after surgery and may resolve with simple drainage and antibiotics. On the other hand, if the abscess or fistula is from Crohn's disease, more than likely it will occur months to years after surgery and will probably require more intensive

Anastomotic leak
breakdown of the anastomosis, usually caused by an infection, in which intestinal bacteria leak out and cause an even worse infection.

therapy to heal. Recurrent abscesses and fistulas, especially a pouch-vaginal fistula, are also suggestive of Crohn's disease.

Female fertility has been reported to be markedly reduced after ileal pouch surgery. One study found a 38.1% infertility rate in 153 patients with ulcerative colitis after pouch surgery, as compared with an infertility rate of 13.3% in 60 patients with ulcerative colitis that were treated medically. Male impotence and retrograde ejaculation has also been reported in approximately 2% of men after they have had ileal pouch surgery.

Finally, fecal incontinence has been reported to occur in up to half of all patients after ileal pouch surgery. Often, this can be treated with antidiarrheal drugs and bulking agents, such as Metamucil, Fibercon, and Konsyl.

PART SEVEN

Diet and Nutrition

I find that if I watch what I eat and eliminate certain foods, I feel better. Does that mean that Crohn's disease and ulcerative colitis are caused by something in the diet and can be cured by eating the right types of food?

Is IBD caused by a food allergy?

Is there a specific diet that I should follow if I have Crohn's disease or ulcerative colitis?

More...

53. I find that if I watch what I eat and eliminate certain foods, I feel better. Does that mean that Crohn's disease and ulcerative colitis are caused by something in the diet and can be cured by eating the right types of food?

The causes of Crohn's disease and ulcerative colitis are not known, but it is believed they are not related to diet. This is not to say that diet does not play a role in IBD—it does. What you eat always has an impact on how you feel. Limiting your diet to foods that do not cause intestinal upset would make anyone feel better. This type of dietary modification is helpful for any type of intestinal problem, not just for IBD. What is clear is that in Crohn's disease and ulcerative colitis, modifying your diet does not have an effect on the actual underlying inflammation. Dietary modification, however, does have an effect on the symptoms. For example, patients with Crohn's disease who have intestinal strictures are less likely to experience a bowel obstruction if they avoid foods that are hard to digest fully, such as raw fruit and vegetables, nuts and berries, corn, and even popcorn. Or, as another example, a patient with ulcerative colitis who has diarrhea should avoid caffeine-containing beverages, such as coffee, tea, and soda, because they are known to worsen diarrhea. Many patients report improvement in their IBD symptoms simply after they stop eating at fast-food restaurants. So, although IBD is not caused by anything in the diet, paying attention to what you eat can still help you feel better.

What you eat always has an impact on how you feel.

114

Ken's comment:

I've learned over time what foods I can and can't eat. Even when my ulcerative colitis is in remission, certain foods cause cramping, gas, and general discomfort. Hot dogs are out, asparagus is a no-no, and I've pretty much cut fast food out of my diet entirely. It can be hard sometimes to avoid the foods that I know will cause me some discomfort, like at barbeques or sporting events, but with a little planning ahead I can usually get by. I always keep in mind that no matter how good that hot dog might look, do I really want to pay the price later?

Jennifer's comment:

Through what some might consider painful trial and error, I have discovered that the foods I eat (as well as those that I avoid) play a big role in how I feel.

When my Crohn's is active, roughage of any kind—mainly raw vegetables and fruit—is the enemy. These types of food tend to significantly exacerbate the Crohn's symptoms that I might be experiencing at the time. Needless to say, I steer clear of these foods when experiencing acute flare-ups.

In contrast, when in remission, I can eat just about anything, including raw vegetables and fruit, without the painful consequences. However, for some reason, greasy, fried food (the kind you find at popular fast-food restaurants) as well as broccoli (a former favorite of mine) send my intestinal tract into a tailspin, even on my healthiest days. As a result, I tend to avoid these types of food because the side effects, in my opinion, are not worth the few minutes of enjoyment.

Despite my good intentions to eat healthy, I have difficulty resisting some temptations. For example, my body does tolerate caffeine, but not well enough for me to avoid some mild side effects (i.e., occasional diarrhea). Rather than give up my morning coffee habit, however, I am willing to accept the consequences of my actions.

Food choices have neither triggered nor eradicated the symptoms of my Crohn's disease. However, smart dietary choices have allowed me to better control how I feel on a daily basis.

No scientific evidence links Crohn's disease or ulcerative colitis to food allergies.

54. Is IBD caused by a food allergy?

No. No scientific evidence links Crohn's disease or ulcerative colitis to food allergies. The vast majority of adults who believe that they have an allergy to food are actually suffering from **food intolerance**, or intolerance to the method by which the food is prepared. The difference between **food allergy** and food intolerance is that a food allergy is caused by an immune system reaction, whereas intolerance does not involve the immune system. Lactose intolerance is a common example of a food intolerance. Allergies to tree nuts, peanuts, cow's milk, eggs, soy, fish, and shellfish are the most common true food allergies. Children often outgrow allergies to cow's milk, eggs, and soy. Those who are allergic to tree nuts, peanuts, fish, and shellfish usually remain allergic for life.

What should you do if you believe you are intolerant of a certain food? The most obvious measure is to eliminate that food from your diet and see if you feel better. Common sense dictates that if a food doesn't agree with you, avoid it! As mentioned earlier, certain foods are best avoided during a flare of Crohn's disease or ulcerative colitis. So, although many people often wonder whether gastrointestinal diseases are related to true food allergies, few, if any, are.

55. How does having Crohn's disease or ulcerative colitis affect my nutrition?

Most of the food that you eat is broken down in the stomach and absorbed in the small intestine. Many disorders can affect the small intestine and interfere with its ability to absorb nutrients properly. When this occurs, it is called malabsorption. The nutrients that may be malabsorbed include a wide variety of food breakdown products such as carbohydrates, fats, and proteins. Other essential dietary elements can also be affected, including iron, calcium, zinc, vitamin B_{12}, folate, and the fat-soluble vitamins A, D, E, and K.

Malabsorption can cause a variety of symptoms. If severe, it can cause weight loss, fatigue, and diarrhea. The diarrhea is often described as foul smelling, with greasy stools that may float in the toilet bowl, become difficult to flush, and leave an "oil slick" on the surface of the water. These changes in stool are often caused by malabsorption of fat, which can be measured in the stool. Again, these types of symptoms are often found only in the later stages of severe malabsorption. Most individuals with malabsorption may have only mild symptoms or no symptoms at all. Sometimes the only sign of malabsorption is the presence of anemia or a vitamin deficiency.

Malabsorption can cause a variety of symptoms.

Individuals with Crohn's disease that involves the small bowel often have some level of malabsorption, whether it is obvious by symptoms or shows up only on blood tests.

Individuals with Crohn's disease that involves the small bowel often have some level of malabsorption, whether it is obvious by symptoms or shows up only on blood tests. This is because over time inflammation of the small bowel can cause damage to the intestinal lining, which interferes with the absorption of food products. Your gastroenterologist is always on the lookout for signs of malabsorption and may order blood tests routinely to ensure that you do not develop major vitamin or nutrient deficiencies. Patients with Crohn's disease can develop anemia caused by iron, folate, or B_{12} deficiencies. Two other very important nutrients are calcium and vitamin D. Malabsorption of these nutrients, which can potentially lead to osteoporosis, can be found in individuals with small bowel Crohn's disease or anyone with IBD who takes long-term corticosteroids (see Question 56).

Short gut syndrome

a condition of severe malabsorption caused by extensive small bowel resection.

Individuals who have had portions of their small bowel surgically removed may suffer from malabsorption because of the simple fact that there is less small bowel available for absorption of nutrients. If enough small bowel is removed, patients can develop short bowel syndrome (also called **short gut syndrome**). This is mostly seen in patients who have had Crohn's disease for many years and who have had multiple surgeries from which less than 100 cm of small bowel remains. These individuals have a very tough time keeping up with absorption of food and fluids, and they can easily become malnourished or dehydrated.

Patients who have short bowel often need additional intravenous nutrition in the form of total parenteral nutrition, or **TPN**. TPN is administered on a daily basis through a permanent IV line that is surgically placed into a deep vein to allow for a high concentration of nutrients to be administered; small, superficial veins, such as those on the hands and arms, are too frail to withstand the daily infusion of highly concentrated nutrition. Patients are taught to self-administer TPN at home, usually over 10 to 12 hours at night. Nationwide companies exist solely to provide home nutrition and employ teams of nurses and medical assistants specially trained to provide the necessary support right in your home. If you are on home TPN and want to go on vacation, the "bags" of TPN can be delivered wherever you go. Although this may sound drastic, individuals on long-term home TPN can live happy, healthy, and independent lives. For example, one patient on home TPN even goes skydiving!

Ulcerative colitis does not affect the small intestine and, therefore, does not cause malabsorption. However, someone with ulcerative colitis can become malnourished if he or she is ill with severe colitis and as a result has not been eating enough. The same holds true for someone with active Crohn's colitis who may have an intact and normally functioning small bowel but who can still become malnourished because of a reduced food intake to avoid exacerbating symptoms.

Ulcerative colitis does not affect the small intestine and, therefore, does not cause malabsorption.

What is the difference between malabsorption and **malnutrition**? As stated earlier, malabsorption occurs when the small intestine loses its ability to absorb the nutrients and vitamins from the food that you eat. Malnutrition is an end result of malabsorption, when your body is unable to take in enough nutrients to maintain good health. Malnutrition can also happen if you don't eat enough or eat only junk foods.

56. How do I know if I should take vitamins?

Eating a healthy diet is sage advice for anyone wanting to maintain good health. For individuals with IBD, following this advice can, at times, prove to be challenging. Patients with Crohn's disease and ulcerative colitis often live with dietary restrictions that make it difficult to eat a well-balanced diet. And because vitamins come from the various food groups, eating a restricted diet may reduce the intake of the recommended daily allotment of vitamins. Therefore, anyone who is on a restricted diet should take a daily multivitamin to supplement what he or she may be missing.

Patients with Crohn's disease and ulcerative colitis often live with dietary restrictions that make it difficult to eat a well–balanced diet.

Selective vitamin deficiencies can also occur in IBD. This is more commonly found in people with small bowel Crohn's disease than it is in colonic Crohn's disease or ulcerative colitis because absorption of vitamins occurs mostly in the small bowel. Vitamin B_{12} is absorbed in the ileum. Accordingly, vitamin B_{12} deficiency can be found in individuals with ileal Crohn's disease or after an ileal resection. Because the deficiency is not caused by a lack of dietary vitamin B_{12}, but rather from an inability to absorb vitamin B_{12}, oral supplementation with vitamin B_{12} tablets is not effective. In this setting, vitamin B_{12} must be given through a different route—as a monthly injection or a weekly application of nasal gel. Calcium and vitamin D deficiency are also commonly seen in Crohn's disease, both from reduced dietary intake and decreased absorption. These deficiencies usually can be treated with calcium and vitamin D tablets. Zinc deficiency may also be found in Crohn's disease and should be supplemented with zinc tablets. Folic acid deficiency can occur in patients taking sulfasalazine because of sulfasalazine's interference with the normal absorption of folic acid. For this reason, all patients taking sulfasalazine should also be on a daily folic acid supplement.

Iron deficiency is commonly found both in Crohn's disease and ulcerative colitis. Usually resulting from intestinal blood loss caused by active IBD, it can also be the result of reduced dietary intake and, in Crohn's disease, decreased absorption. In addition to treating the active IBD, often patients are also given an oral iron supplement. Patients who are unable to tolerate oral iron, which may cause gastrointestinal side effects, can be given intravenous iron instead. Magnesium deficiency as a result of intestinal losses can be seen in patients with chronic diarrhea and can be supplemented with magnesium oxide. Trace element deficiency is rare and is found only in individuals who have had extensive small bowel resection and those who are usually on home parenteral nutrition.

A common question is whether you should take any particular brand of vitamins given that many vitamins are marketed specifically for IBD patients and are purported to be better than typical over-the-counter vitamins. The answer is no. The vitamins you can get in any drug store are usually equal to any of the more expensive vitamins that are marketed to IBD patients. You need not spend more money on brand names when the generic vitamins are equally as good.

57. I'm chronically underweight. What can I do to gain weight?

Because of dietary restrictions, patients with Crohn's disease and ulcerative colitis often find it difficult to maintain their ideal body weight. Whereas the majority of Americans are overweight and are constantly dieting, not infrequently individuals with IBD find themselves on the lower end of the scale trying to climb back up. There is no trick to gaining weight— eat more calories. However, when you have Crohn's disease or ulcerative colitis, this is easier said than done. First, if you are underweight, you should take a daily multivitamin and be checked to see if you have any particular vitamin deficiencies that need to be corrected. Next, rather than trying to gorge yourself at breakfast, lunch, and dinner, which can leave you feeling overfilled, uncomfortable, and possibly with worsening IBD symptoms, you should instead try eating small but frequent meals. The meals should consist of nutritional and high-caloric foods. Desserts and snacks in between meals are encouraged. Although you should never force yourself to eat, you should also not deny yourself food whenever you are hungry. Last, if this is not enough to allow you to gain the desired amount of weight, nutritional supplements, such as Carnation Instant Breakfast, Ensure, or Boost, for example, are often helpful.

In addition to adding calories, moderate exercise with light weightlifting can also assist you in gaining

There is no trick to gaining weight— eat more calories. However, when you have Crohn's disease or ulcerative colitis, this is easier said than done.

weight. However, strenuous aerobic exercise can lead to further weight loss, so avoid this.

58. Since I have to avoid fruits and vegetables due to my Crohn's disease, what can I do to lose weight?

Having to follow a restricted diet, particularly having to avoid fruits and vegetables, poses particular difficulties for those who are challenged by being overweight. The traditional program of diet and exercise is still the cornerstone for weight loss. Especially if your diet is restricted because of Crohn's disease or ulcerative colitis, regular exercise is of paramount importance. Vigorous aerobic exercise expends the greatest amount of energy and, therefore, can likely lead to weight loss. However, even low-intensity exercise, such as walking or climbing stairs, is beneficial. Multiple repetitions of lifting light weights also helps you lose weight. Heavy weightlifting, on the other hand, may result in weight gain, although heavy lifting may assist in losing fat and gaining muscle.

Most diets designed to help you lose weight consist of increasing the proportion of low-caloric foods, such as fresh fruits and vegetables, and reducing the proportion of high-caloric/high-fat (especially saturated fat) foods, such as fried foods, desserts, and snacks. For patients with Crohn's disease and ulcerative colitis, a diet high in fresh fruits and vegetables often causes worsening symptoms and, therefore, is avoided.

So, what can an IBD patient eat and lose weight? A high-protein, low-fat diet (i.e., modified Atkins diet)

The traditional program of diet and exercise is still the cornerstone for weight loss. Especially if your diet is restricted because of Crohn's disease or ulcerative colitis, regular exercise is of paramount importance.

is usually well tolerated and palatable. Along with regular exercise, this approach, if you follow it consistently, usually leads to sustained weight loss.

Caveat: Anyone on prednisone will find it difficult to lose weight because of fluid retention and hyperphagia—the need to constantly eat. Avoiding salt helps in reducing fluid retention.

59. What foods should I eat or avoid if I have chronic diarrhea?

Diarrhea is one of the most frustrating and embarrassing symptoms of Crohn's disease and ulcerative colitis. Treating the underlying IBD is critical in managing chronic diarrhea; dietary modification can also be helpful. Certain dietary substances are known to cause diarrhea. Caffeine, coffee, and tea act as stimulants that can "rev up" the bowel and result in diarrhea. Fresh fruits and uncooked vegetables, high-fiber foods such as fiber-rich breads and cereals, and, at times, dairy products may also exacerbate diarrhea. Ice-cold liquids, even water, can cause cramps and diarrhea as well. In fact, too much of any type of liquid can lead to excess bowel movements. Glucose and electrolyte-based drinks, such as Gatorade and Crystal Light, especially when diluted with water, are usually easier to absorb. Foods that may help solidify bowel movements include bananas, white bread, white rice, and cheese (if you're not lactose intolerant).

Treating the underlying IBD is critical in managing chronic diarrhea; dietary modification can also be helpful.

60. What foods should I eat or avoid if I have a stricture?

An intestinal stricture, or narrowing, is a partial blockage of the bowel that is commonly found in Crohn's disease. A stricture can develop from active intestinal inflammation, leftover scarring from prior inflammation, or a combination of the two. Small bowel strictures are best diagnosed with an upper GI small bowel series, whereas colonic strictures are more easily seen with a barium enema or colonoscopy.

Because the intestine is narrowed, much like a pipe with a clog in it, certain foods may not pass through easily. Fortunately, because most food is digested and absorbed in the upper small bowel and most strictures in Crohn's disease occur in the lower small bowel, many patients do not know that they have a stricture. However, certain foods that are difficult to digest can travel undigested down through the intestinal tract and eventually block the stricture (see Question 36). Usually, this is a transient event, and you might experience abdominal pain and distention that lasts anywhere from 30 minutes to a few hours shortly after you finish a meal. At other times, the blockage persists and you might experience severe abdominal pain, distention, vomiting, and might not be able to pass **flatus** (gas) or have a bowel movement. In these most severe cases, you need to be hospitalized for treatment.

You should avoid foods that are difficult to digest and, as a result, are more likely to cause a blockage. These include fresh fruit and raw vegetables, nuts and berries, corn and popcorn, and the less tender cuts of beef. As a rule of thumb, if what you are about to eat requires a lot of chewing, you probably shouldn't eat it.

Foods that are less fibrous are better to eat so you can avoid a blockage. These include fish, pasta, ground beef, small pieces of chicken, thoroughly cooked vegetables, rice, potatoes, eggs, cheese, most breads, most desserts, and soft fruits such as bananas.

Each individual will have to learn which foods his or her body can tolerate and which foods he or she should avoid.

61. Is there a specific diet that I should follow if I have Crohn's disease or ulcerative colitis?

Good nutri-tion not only helps your body function at its best, but also promotes a strong immune sys-tem and a pos-itive sense of well-being.

Nutrition is an important part of everyday life. Good nutrition not only helps your body function at its best, but also promotes a strong immune system and a posi-tive sense of well-being. This becomes more true for patients with Crohn's disease and ulcerative colitis. Naturally, everyone should strive to eat a healthy, bal-anced diet, especially those who have IBD. This said, there is no specific diet you should follow, unless cer-tain foods have made your symptoms worse (see Ques-tions 59 and 60).

*The **specific carbohydrate diet** is a grain-free, lactose-free, sucrose-free diet intended for patients with IBD and has also been suggested for patients with IBS, celiac disease, and diverticulitis.*

The "specific carbohydrate diet" has been proposed by some as a good diet for patients with Crohn's disease and ulcerative colitis. The **specific carbohydrate diet** is a grain-free, lactose-free, sucrose-free diet intended for patients with IBD and has also been suggested for patients with IBS, celiac disease, and diverticulitis. The theory behind this diet is that carbohydrates (sug-ars) in a normal diet act as fuel for the overgrowth of bacteria and yeast in the small intestine. This over-growth can cause an imbalance that damages the lin-ing of the small intestine and impairs its ability to digest and absorb all nutrients, including carbohy-drates. The excess of unabsorbed carbohydrates further fuels the vicious cycle of overgrowth and imbalance.

Promoters of this diet also believe that harmful toxins are produced by the excess bacteria and yeast inhabiting the small intestine.

By consuming only certain types of carbohydrates, people using this diet hope to eliminate bacterial and yeast overgrowth. Believers claim up to an 80% recovery rate in patients with Crohn's disease and an even higher "cure" rate in patients with problems such as IBS and diverticulitis. Following are certain food guidelines for the specific carbohydrate diet.

Foods to avoid:

- Canned vegetables
- Canned fruits, unless they are packed in their own juices
- All cereal grains, including flour
- Potatoes, yams, parsnips, chickpeas, bean sprouts, soybeans, mung beans, fava beans, and seaweed
- Processed meats, breaded or canned fish, processed cheeses, smoked or canned meat
- Milk or dried milk solids
- Buttermilk or acidophilus milk, commercially prepared yogurt and sour cream, soy milk, instant tea or coffee, coffee substitutes, and beer
- Cornstarch, arrowroot or other starches, chocolate or carob, bouillon cubes or instant soup bases, all products made with refined sugar, agar-agar, carrageenan or pectin, ketchup, ice cream, molasses, corn or maple syrup, flours made from legumes, baking powder, medication containing sugar, and all seeds

Foods to eat:

- Fresh and frozen vegetables and legumes
- Fresh, raw, or dried fruits
- Fresh or frozen meats, poultry, fish, and eggs
- Natural cheeses, homemade yogurt, and dry curd cottage cheese

Although this diet may seem like a simple, natural way to treat Crohn's disease, it has yet to be proved scientifically to help people with IBD. Although the "Foods to eat" list provides a healthy alternative to many items on the "Foods to avoid" list, several comments need to made about the diet as a whole. First and foremost, special diets should never be used as treatments for IBD and should never replace medications that you have found to be beneficial. Although healthy diet choices should be a part of everyone's lifestyle, eliminating too many foods from a diet can be cumbersome. Patients who may also be lactose intolerant should avoid milk products. Also, fresh foods are a healthier alternative to canned or processed foods. However, during an IBD flare, too many fresh fruits and vegetables can create a big fiber load for the small intestine and colon (Question 59). The bottom line is beware of special diets that make big promises.

62. Do all patients with Crohn's disease or ulcerative colitis have lactose intolerance?

Lactose intolerance is a very common problem for many people. It is caused by a deficiency of the **lactase** enzyme, which is found in the small intestine. Lactose is a major ingredient in dairy products such as milk, ice cream, yogurt, and cheese. There are also many less obvious sources of lactose. Did you know lactose can even be found in certain pills and deli meats? Some nutritional supplements such as Ensure, even though they may look like a milkshake, do not contain lactose.

Symptoms of lactose intolerance include diarrhea, bloating, flatulence, and abdominal cramps after ingesting a lactose-containing product. The only two treatments are lactose avoidance or taking supplemental lactase enzymes (such as Lactaid) before eating or drinking a dairy product. Remember that if you are lactose intolerant, you'll need to find other ways to supplement your calcium and vitamin D intake because you will no longer be getting them from your diet.

Because the lactase enzyme is found in the small intestine, individuals with Crohn's disease may also be prone to lactose intolerance as a result of inflammation and damage to the lining of the small intestine, which interfere with lactose absorption. Even healthy patients who get a "stomach bug" or viral gastroenteritis can have problems digesting lactose products for a little while until the lining of the bowels can heal. It is reasonable to eliminate dairy from your diet for a week or 2 after a diarrheal illness until the level of lactase enzyme can return to normal.

There are two ways to diagnose lactose intolerance. The most common way is to avoid dairy for 1 week and see if the cramps and diarrhea go away. Then drink a glass of milk and see if they recur. If you still are not sure whether you are lactose intolerant, your doctor can order a **lactose breath test** as a more objective measurement. Sugars (such as lactose) not absorbed properly in the small intestine make their way to the colon where they are metabolized by bacteria. These bacteria give off hydrogen, which quickly crosses the lining of the colon into the bloodstream and can be measured in the breath.

The day before the lactose breath test, you are instructed to avoid high-fiber foods that can cause an unusually high baseline level of hydrogen in the initial breath samples. Brushing your teeth also helps to decrease excess bacteria in your mouth that can also cause abnormally high baseline hydrogen readings. At the start of the test, you blow into the machine and the hydrogen level is measured. Then, you are instructed to drink a solution that has a high amount of lactose. Subsequent breath measurements for hydrogen are taken at 15- to 30-minute intervals over a 2-hour period. The total rise in hydrogen from the baseline measurement is then calculated. If this rise is greater than 20 parts per minute (ppm), lactose intolerance may be present. Certain situations such as recent antibiotic use, gastroenteritis, or small bowel bacterial overgrowth can cause the results to be inaccurate.

PART EIGHT

Extraintestinal Manifestations

Can IBD affect parts of my body other than just my bowels?

My joints are often stiff and sore. Is this related to my IBD?

Am I more likely to get osteoporosis if I have Crohn's disease or ulcerative colitis?

More ...

63. Can IBD affect parts of my body other than just my bowels?

Crohn's disease and ulcerative colitis can affect many different parts of your body (see Table 11). These are referred to as the *extraintestinal manifestations* of IBD because these effects are found outside of the gastrointestinal tract. Extraintestinal manifestations are also called **systemic** because they reflect a process involving the body as whole, as opposed to *local* symptoms, which occur just in the intestinal tract. Systemic symptoms include fatigue, weight loss, anemia, and sometimes low-grade fevers. Extraintestinal manifestations

Table 11   Extraintestinal Manifestations of Crohn's Disease and Ulcerative Colitis

Common
Joint pains
Skin rashes
Mouth ulcers
Gallstones
Liver disease (PSC)
Eye problems
Growth retardation in children

Uncommon
Anemia
Blood clots
Kidney stones
Nerve damage
Lung disease
Pancreatitis (inflammation of the pancreas)
Pericarditis (inflammation around the heart)

PSC, Primary sclerosing cholangitis.

can also be more localized to a specific organ. Organs that can be affected include the skin, eyes, joints, bones, kidneys, urinary tract, reproductive system, **gallbladder**, liver, and circulatory system. Although this list is quite long, extraintestinal manifestations do not occur in every patient. Approximately 25% of individuals with Crohn's disease and ulcerative colitis may develop one or more of the extraintestinal manifestations. Joint symptoms, such as arthritis, are the most common and are often seen together with skin and eye symptoms. Extraintestinal manifestations are found more often in individuals with ulcerative colitis or in individuals with Crohn's disease that primarily affects the colon; they are seen less often with predominantly small bowel disease.

We do not yet know what causes extraintestinal manifestations to develop, just as we do not know the cause of Crohn's disease or ulcerative colitis. The leading theory is that because IBD is believed to be a result of a defect in the immune system, this same defect could potentially lead to inflammation in other areas of the body in addition to the gastrointestinal tract. Why certain people develop extraintestinal manifestations and others do not is a mystery.

The presence of extraintestinal manifestations often provides additional clues as to the level of activity of the underlying IBD. This is because, in many cases, extraintestinal manifestations often reflect ongoing intestinal inflammation that may not be apparent to either you or your physician. In fact, some individuals use their extraintestinal manifestations as a signal as to when they are about to have a flare. One particular patient, for

The presence of extraintestinal manifestations often provides additional clues as to the level of activity of the underlying IBD.

example, calls her physician and states that in a few days she will have a flare of her ulcerative colitis—she knows this because she always has an ulcerative colitis flare after she notices a certain type of skin rash.

In general, effective treatment of the underlying IBD usually leads to resolution of the extraintestinal symptoms. Some of the extraintestinal manifestations, however, run a course independent from the underlying IBD and do not improve along with improvements in the intestinal symptoms (more about this later). It is also important to remember that systemic symptoms are sometimes a result of a drug-induced side effect and not from an extraintestinal manifestation.

Now you know why your doctor asks a long list of questions concerning many aspects of your overall health and does not focus just on your bowels at each visit. Crohn's disease and ulcerative colitis involve not just the gastrointestinal tract, but can affect many different areas of the body as well. Indeed, at times the extraintestinal manifestations can be severe enough to overshadow a person's underlying intestinal symptoms. It is for this reason that you should inform your doctor when you are having new symptoms, even if they seem unrelated to your bowel disease.

64. How can IBD affect my skin?

The two most common types of skin rashes seen in individuals with Crohn's disease and ulcerative colitis are **erythema nodosum** and **pyoderma gangrenosum**. Both rashes are very distinctive. Erythema nodosum appears as a painful, tender, reddish-purplish bump that occurs mostly on the shins; it can be found over the rest of the legs and arms as well. Erythema nodosum is a sign that your IBD is active. With treatment of the bowel disease, this rash should go away.

Unlike erythema nodosum, pyoderma gangrenosum can appear at any time and is not related to the activity of the underlying intestinal inflammation. Pyoderma gangrenosum is found most commonly on the legs and adjacent to an ileostomy or colostomy, although it can appear anywhere on your body. It starts as a red, inflamed area of skin usually smaller than the size of a dime. This inflamed area soon forms a punched-out, sharply demarcated ulcer with a raised reddish-purplish border. Pyoderma gangrenosum exhibits what is called the ***pathergy phenomenon***. This is an unusual dermatologic condition in which a skin ulcer can get bigger and deeper as a result of even minor trauma, such as abrasive cleaning or pulling off a sticky dressing. For this reason, you should never attempt surgery on pyoderma gangrenosum. Because of the pathergy phenomenon, it can get large enough so that it takes months to heal. Pyoderma gangrenosum is not a common rash and, therefore, can be difficult to diagnose by the untrained eye. Any individual with Crohn's disease or ulcerative colitis who develops an ulcer on the skin should be considered to have pyoderma gangrenosum until it is proved otherwise.

Several treatments are available for pyoderma gangrenosum. First and foremost, the ulcer should be bandaged with a nonstick dressing so as to avoid trauma when you change the dressing. First-line therapy usually consists of topical therapy with a corticosteroid ointment and cromolyn sodium. Topical cyclosporine (Protopic) has also shown good results. Corticosteroids can also be injected directly into the ulcer, but this approach is limited to use only on small ulcers and is not used as often as topical therapy. If topical therapy and/or corticosteroid injection is not successful, systemic therapy with oral or IV corticosteroids and various immune-modulating drugs, such as infliximab (Remicade) and cyclosporine, have been found to be beneficial. In addition, even though pyoderma gangrenosum may occur in an individual whose IBD is in remission, it can also appear in someone with active IBD. In such a case, the active inflammation should be treated aggressively.

65. I often get little sores in my mouth, especially when my IBD is active. Are these related, and what can I do about them?

Sometimes IBD patients can develop small, painful sores in the mouth called **apthous ulcers**. They can be very bothersome and appear much like canker sores. Infrequently, much larger ulcers can develop. Topical oral anesthetics, such as lidocaine, can be helpful to numb the pain. A topical corticosteroid is often mixed in with the anesthetic. Usually the oral ulcers occur when the intestinal inflammation has become more active. Mouth sores can also develop as a side effect of some of the medications used to treat IBD. Antibiotics, for example, can cause **thrush**, which is an oral fungal infection. Also, the immune-modulating drugs can leave your body susceptible to viral infections such as the herpes simplex virus (HSV) or cytomegalovirus (CMV), both of which can cause sores on the lips and inside the mouth. Finally, Crohn's disease can directly affect the mouth. In these cases, the findings can range from multiple, small aphothous ulcers to large, irregular ulcers. Crohn's disease can also cause severe **gingivitis**. Last, *pyostomatitis vege-tans* is a rare oral manifestation of Crohn's disease. Often considered to be an oral presentation of pyoderma gangrenosum, multiple small pustules, ulcers, and abscesses occur in the oral cavity. They can be treated with topical and oral corticosteroids as well as immune-modulating drugs.

66. My joints are often stiff and sore. Is this related to my IBD?

Individuals with Crohn's disease or ulcerative colitis often complain of having sore and stiff joints. The medical term for soreness and stiffness in the joints is arthralgia. Arthritis is when the joints are actually inflamed—painful, red, swollen, and warm. These IBD-associated joint symptoms can be divided into two categories: those that affect the central or spinal joints (back, pelvis, hips), and those that affect the peripheral joints (shoulders, elbows, wrists, fingers, knees, ankles, toes).

Peripheral arthralgias may be seen in up to 30% of individuals with Crohn's disease and ulcerative colitis. These patients often experience painful, stiff joints throughout their body. A single joint or several joints can be affected at the same time, or the pain can migrate from one joint to another. Sometimes a true arthritis can be seen with a red, hot, and swollen joint. IBD-associated arthritis is different from both **osteoarthritis** (so-called wear-and-tear arthritis) and rheumatoid arthritis; IBD-associated arthritis in a nondestructive form of arthritis, meaning that it does not permanently damage the joints. Conversely, the other forms of arthritis do lead to joint destruction. For this reason, it is important for your doctor to investigate any new joint symptoms you have because they may be caused by a variety of illnesses. If a single joint is red, hot, or swollen, it could mean the joint is infected. **Gout** is another condition that can cause pain in a single joint, often the big toe. In gout, uric acid crystals form and become concentrated in the joint fluid, causing inflammation and pain. Your doctor may want to remove a sample of fluid from the joint with a small needle to send for laboratory analysis and examination under a microscope to rule out these other causes of joint pain.

Peripheral arthralgias associated with Crohn's disease and ulcerative colitis usually mirror the activity of the underlying bowel disease. In other words, the joint pains probably develop as a result of active IBD. Accordingly, treatment of underlying bowel symptoms usually makes the joint pains feel better.

Central (spinal) arthralgias occur in approximately 5% of people with Crohn's disease or ulcerative colitis. The joints that are most affected include those of the lower spine and pelvis, specifically the sacroiliac joints within the pelvis. Patients may develop pain or stiffness in the lower back that is worse in the morning upon waking and improves with activity throughout the day. Unlike peripheral arthritis, arthritis affecting the central joints can lead to permanent damage, when joints fuse together in the vertebral column, as well as in the sacroiliac region. Central arthritis is also different from peripheral arthritis in that it is not necessarily associated with the level of bowel activity. In fact, central arthritis can show up years before bowel symptoms occur. Treatment of bowel symptoms does not help this type of arthritis. Rather, treatment is targeted toward helping control the arthritis symptoms. Range of motion exercises, physical therapy, and moist heat applied to the back can be helpful.

Jennifer's comment:

I developed an IBD-related arthritic pain in my right hip within a year or so after my first bowel resection. Although sporadic in its occurrence, when the pain is at its worst, I experience stiffness and a throbbing ache in that joint area. During these episodes, my joint symptoms are exacerbated when I put weight on my right leg.

I have not been able to identify a trigger or consistent pattern for these painful occurrences. At times it seems this pain coincides with a change (for the worse) in the weather or when I'm fighting a cold or virus that has settled in my intestinal tract. At other times, however, my hip aches when I'm in "perfect" health and when the sun is shining.

A series of X rays has not detected any deterioration of that particular joint over the years, and I have long given up trying to make sense of this unusual side effect of my disease. I typically alleviate these aches and pains with an over-the-counter pain reliever as well as extra rest, which usually includes time on the couch to keep undue pressure off my hip. I have also found acupuncture to be a very effective treatment for these joint symptoms. Regardless, these therapies have proved temporary because this joint pain has become a permanent aspect of my disease.

67. Are any of the drugs that treat IBD also helpful in treating the joint pains?

Nonsteroidal anti-inflammatory drugs (NSAIDs) are the most commonly used drugs to treat joint pains. These medications include ibuprofen (Advil, Motrin), naproxen (Aleve), and celecoxib (Celebrex). Although these drugs are effective in treating the pain and inflammation, they can also lead to a flare of Crohn's disease or ulcerative colitis. For this reason, IBD patients should avoid taking these drugs on a regular basis. Acetaminophen (Tylenol), on the other hand, is okay to use in Crohn's disease or ulcerative colitis.

As mentioned in the previous question, peripheral arthralgias can improve with effective treatment of the underlying bowel disease. Certain medications used in the treatment of Crohn's disease and ulcerative colitis work better on joint symptoms than others do.

Sulfasalazine was originally developed in the 1930s to treat rheumatoid arthritis. It was later found to be beneficial in ulcerative colitis, and then Crohn's colitis, as well. Still used by rheumatologists to treat arthritis, sulfasalazine is a good drug to use in patients with Crohn's disease or ulcerative colitis and joint pain.

Prednisone is a potent anti-inflammatory drug commonly used to treat IBD as well as arthritis. Individuals with Crohn's disease and ulcerative colitis who also have IBD-associated arthritis find that using prednisone rapidly improves their joint symptoms along with their bowel disease.

Methotrexate is used frequently in the treatment of arthritis. Although not used very often for Crohn's disease, it is a reasonable choice for someone with both active Crohn's disease and arthritic complaints.

Infliximab has been shown to be an effective treatment for Crohn's disease, ulcerative colitis, and arthritis. It is an excellent choice for patients with Crohn's disease or ulcerative colitis who also have IBD-associated arthritis.

68. How do I know if I am at risk for osteoporosis, and is there any way to prevent it?

Osteoporosis is a disease in which the bones are severely weakened as result of a loss of bone density. Osteoporosis is a silent disease that can be diagnosed, treated, and prevented. Millions of Americans are at risk (see Table 12), and women are four times as likely as men to develop osteoporosis. The most serious complications include fractures of the spine and hips and can lead to significant loss of independence. Risks for osteoporosis include female gender, advanced age, small or thin body size, fair-skinned, and a family history of osteoporosis. Unfortunately, most people have no control over these risk factors. Certain lifestyle choices can promote healthy bones, such as quitting smoking, avoiding excessive alcohol intake, exercising regularly with weight-bearing activities (walking, lifting weights), and eating a diet rich in calcium and vitamin D.

Millions of Americans are at risk, and women are four times as likely as men to develop osteoporosis.

Table 12   Risk Factors for Osteoporosis

Female gender
Advanced age
Small or thin body size
Fair skin
Family history of osteoporosis
Cigarette smoking
Excess alcohol
Prolonged use of corticosteroids
Crohn's disease

The recommended daily allowance of calcium is 1000 to 1500 milligrams a day, and vitamin D is 400 to 800 international units (IU) a day. Dairy products contain excellent amounts of calcium and vitamin D, including milk, cheese, yogurt, and ice cream. Tofu, almonds, and dark green leafy vegetables such as spinach, bok choy, collard greens, and broccoli are also good sources of calcium. Some foods such as breads and orange juice are now fortified with calcium and/or vitamin D. Individuals who are lactose intolerant or feel they do not get enough calcium and vitamin D in their diets can take oral supplements. These can be purchased over the counter in grocery stores and pharmacies, and often contain combinations of calcium and vitamin D in one pill. Calcium *carbonate* preparations need to be taken with food for full effect, whereas calcium *gluconate* pills do not.

69. Am I more likely to get osteoporosis if I have Crohn's disease or ulcerative colitis?

Individuals with Crohn's disease and ulcerative colitis are particularly prone to developing osteoporosis.

Individuals with Crohn's disease and ulcerative colitis are particularly prone to developing osteoporosis. Some studies show loss of bone density in up to 60% of patients. Several potential reasons for this exist. Inflammation of the small bowel in Crohn's disease can lead to poor absorption of calcium and vitamin D, nutrients that are vital for bone health. Along the same lines, because of active IBD, individuals with Crohn's disease and ulcerative colitis often eat less to avoid aggravating their symptoms. They may eat fewer foods containing calcium and vitamin D, such as dairy products. Also, patients with Crohn's disease who have had portions of their small bowel surgically removed may not have enough healthy small bowel remaining to allow for adequate absorption of calcium and vitamin D.

Corticosteroids, one of the mainstays of therapy used to treat Crohn's disease and ulcerative colitis, can cause accelerated bone loss and, with it, premature osteoporosis. The effect of corticosteroids is cumulative, meaning that the higher the dose and the longer time you take a corticosteroid, the greater the likelihood you will develop osteoporosis. If you are taking corticosteroids, it is imperative you make sure you are getting enough calcium and vitamin D either from food or nutritional supplements.

70. How can I tell if I have osteoporosis? Are there ways to treat it?

Osteoporosis can be diagnosed with a bone density scan, which is a specialized X ray used to assess the strength of the bones in the spine and hips. Results of this test are reported in two different ways—the T score and the Z score. The **T score** compares your bone density to that of a young healthy adult with excellent bone density, whereas the **Z score** compares your bone density to a person of the same age, gender, and race. The T score is the result most commonly used by physicians to predict an individual's risk of sustaining a bone fracture as a result of osteoporosis. A T score of greater than −0.9 is normal. A T score of −1.0 to −2.5 indicates a mild loss of bone density, which is a condition called **osteopenia**. Individuals in this category are at double the risk for a bone fracture. A T score of −2.5 or less is defined as osteoporosis. Those with osteoporosis are three to five times more likely to suffer a bone fracture.

If you have osteopenia or osteoporosis, your doctor may decide you should take a medication called a **bisphosphonate**; such as, alendronate sodium (Fosamax) or risedronate sodium (Actonel). This type of medication works together with calcium and vitamin D to slow bone loss. These medications are available in a daily or weekly pill form. Follow directions carefully when you take these medications to avoid side effects, especially irritation to the esophagus. To avoid esophageal irritation, the pills should be taken with a large amount of water while in an upright position (sitting, standing, or walking around) and you should stay upright for at least a half hour after taking the medication.

In addition to taking the preceding medications, avoid the behaviors known to increase the risk of osteoporosis—cigarette smoking, excess alcohol use, and lack of regular weight-bearing exercise—to help strengthen your bones and reduce the risk of fracture.

IBD-associated eye disorders are among the most serious of the extraintestinal manifestations. Left untreated, they can result in permanent damage, including scarring and blindness.

71. Is it true that Crohn's disease and ulcerative colitis can also affect my eyes?

IBD-associated eye disorders are among the most serious of the extraintestinal manifestations. Left untreated, they can result in permanent damage, including scarring and blindness. It is for this reason that you and your physician should be quick to consult an ophthalmologist for prompt diagnosis and treatment of any new **ocular** (i.e., eye) condition. The ophthalmologist will use a slit lamp test (a microscopic view of the inside structures of the eye) to detect different abnormalities. Usually, treatment of the underlying bowel disease can help alleviate the ocular symptoms. Sometimes corticosteroid eye drops are used as well. Regardless, any new ocular symptoms must be evaluated promptly because delay in treatment can cause lasting damage to the eyes.

The three most common eye disorders associated with IBD are **episcleritis**, **iritis**, and **uveitis**. These names are derived from the structures in the eye that have become inflamed. Episcleritis refers to inflammation of the white of the eye; iritis refers to inflammation of the colored part of the eye; and uveitis refers to inflammation of the central portion of the eye (the iris is part of the uvea). Often, the tiny blood vessels of the eye become inflamed, causing them to dilate or expand, which is what causes the eye to become red. Other symptoms include pain, sensitivity to light, and blurred vision. These ocular disorders often occur along with arthritis and erythema nodosum.

Other problems that affect the eyes, such as cataracts and **glaucoma**, can be side effects of the long-term use of corticosteroids. Needing reading glasses as you get older, on the other hand, has nothing to do with Crohn's disease or ulcerative colitis—it's simply part of the natural aging process.

72. I recently developed a kidney stone and my doctor said it was from my IBD. What do Crohn's disease and ulcerative colitis have to do with the kidneys?

Individuals with Crohn's disease and ulcerative colitis are prone to develop kidney stones. The risk of developing a kidney stone is higher with Crohn's disease than with ulcerative colitis, and is also higher in individuals with ileostomies. Just as in the general population, calcium stones are the most common type of

Individuals with Crohn's disease and ulcerative colitis are prone to develop kidney stones.

kidney stone in IBD, although individuals with ileostomies are more likely to get uric acid stones due to diarrhea and dehydration. The primary method to prevent kidney stone formation is by maintaining good hydration and high urine output. Kidney stones are treated by medication, special diets, and by removing the stones.

In addition to kidney stones, the bladder and **ureter** (tube that connects the kidneys to the bladder) can also be affected by Crohn's disease. Fistulas can form between the intestine, mostly the colon, and the bladder or ureter (see Question 40). This can cause recurrent urinary tract infections because the bacteria that live naturally in the colon now have a new route into the urinary tract, which normally is sterile and does not contain bacteria. Urine can also become brown and foul smelling because it is mixed with stool. Individuals with this type of fistula can also experience air coming out when they urinate because gas that is usually in the colon can make its way into the bladder and out through the **urethra** (tunnel that connects the bladder to the outside). Last, Crohn's disease can also cause the ureter to become obstructed, which can lead to **hydronephrosis** (fluid retention in the kidney). This may be seen in cases of severe intestinal inflammation that causes the bowel to swell to the point of impinging on nearby structures, such as the ureter. This can also occur when a stone slips out of the kidney and into the ureter.

73. Are gallstones common in Crohn's disease and ulcerative colitis?

Gallstones are quite common in the general population and can be found in 10–20% of the adult population, although the vast majority of those with gallstones never develop symptoms. Common risk factors for gallstones include female gender, obesity, older age, pregnancy, and certain medications, such as birth control pills. Gallstones can also form after rapid weight loss, such as after obesity surgery. Gallstones are predominantly composed of cholesterol.

Individuals with Crohn's disease involving the terminal ileum may be more prone to the formation of gallstones, although we do not know the exact reason why this happens. One possibility is that gallstones occur because of a disruption in the circulation of bile through the body. Bile is made in the liver and stored in the gallbladder. After you eat, the gallbladder contracts and squirts bile into the intestines where the bile binds to the fats that you have eaten. This complex of bile and fat is then absorbed in the ileum. Ileal inflammation because of Crohn's disease, or removal of the ileum, disrupts the absorption of bile salts. Over time, the bile salts can become depleted, resulting in an imbalance of excess cholesterol and too little bile within the gallbladder, creating the potential for gallstone formation.

One possibility is that gallstones occur because of a disruption in the circulation of bile through the body.

The liver, gallbladder, and pancreas are connected by a network of channels or ducts through which bile and other digestive juices produced in the pancreas flow together and out into the duodenum, the first portion of the small intestine. Gallstones usually form and remain in the gallbladder without causing problems. However, sometimes these stones can become caught in the neck of the gallbladder and cause symptoms as a result of the temporary blockage or obstruction of the gallbladder. This is called **biliary colic**, which refers to intense gallbladder pain caused by spasm. The symptoms of biliary colic may include right-sided upper abdominal pain just under the ribs, nausea, and vomiting. This classically occurs immediately after eating, especially after eating fatty or fried foods. Symptoms can last 30 minutes to hours and go away after the offending gallstone pops back into the gallbladder where it belongs.

Sometimes when a stone gets stuck in the gallbladder, the blockage of bile flow can lead to stagnation and population by bacteria, leading to acute inflammation of the gallbladder, called **cholecystitis**. When this occurs, in addition to biliary colic, patients usually have a fever as well. Occasionally, rather than getting stuck in the gallbladder, a stone can travel out of the gallbladder and get stuck in the bile duct, causing additional symptoms such as **jaundice**, as a result of the backup of bile into the liver. This can also lead to infection of the bile duct, called cholangitis. Individuals who develop cholecystitis or cholangitis often require hospitalization and antibiotics. Once the infection is resolved, surgery is recommended to remove the gallbladder to avoid recurrence of problems. In addition, people who have repeated attacks of biliary colic even in the absence of active blockage or infection should have their gallbladders removed to avoid further symptoms. Individuals who have gallstones stuck in the bile duct may need to have an endoscopic procedure called an ERCP during which the bile duct stones can be removed.

74. How do Crohn's disease and ulcerative colitis affect the liver?

One of the more uncommon extraintestinal manifestations of IBD is primary sclerosing cholangitis (PSC), a disease in which the bile ducts in the liver become narrowed because of inflammation and scarring. Bile is produced by the liver and drains through the bile ducts into the intestines, where it aids digestion. Because in PSC bile cannot drain properly, the bile gets backed up and accumulates in the liver, where it can damage the liver cells. Eventually, the damage can lead to liver cirrhosis and liver failure. At its most extreme, individuals with PSC may end up needing a liver transplantation. Cancer of the bile duct (**cholangiocarcinoma**) can also occur. Individuals with PSC and IBD also have a higher risk of colon cancer than do IBD patients without PSC. The standard recommendation is to perform a surveillance colonoscopy yearly once a patient with ulcerative colitis or Crohn's colitis is diagnosed with PSC.

PSC is seen in fewer than 2% of people with IBD, but as many as 75% of patients with PSC are found to have either Crohn's disease or ulcerative colitis. Usually PSC is associated with ulcerative colitis or Crohn's disease isolated to the colon. Although the cause of PSC is unknown, it is thought that the defect in the immune system that leads to the development of colitis can also affect the liver.

The blockage of bile flow is what causes the signs and symptoms of PSC. Early on, most patients do not have any symptoms. The first sign that something is wrong is usually a rise in one of the liver function tests—the alkaline phosphatase. In fact, most cases of PSC are first discovered with this finding. When symptoms do develop, one of the first is itching of the skin, which is called **pruritus**. Eventually, the patient becomes jaundiced because of an accumulation of bile in the skin and the whites of the eyes. As the bile ducts become progressively scarred, strictures form in

One of the more uncommon extraintestinal manifestations of IBD is primary sclerosing cholangitis (PSC), a disease in which the bile ducts in the liver become narrowed because of inflammation and scarring.

Extraintestinal Manifestations

them. This can lead to an infection of the bile, called cholangitis, in which patients become very ill with fever, chills, jaundice, and tenderness in the right upper abdomen.

PSC is diagnosed by an X ray of the bile ducts, which is called a **cholangiogram**. A cholangiogram can be performed during an endoscopic procedure called an ERCP, or with an MRI of the bile ducts. An ERCP has the advantage of allowing the physician to take samples of the bile for analysis, samples of the strictures to look for cancer, and to dilate, or open up, the strictures to improve the flow of bile. A stent, or small tube, can also be placed through the stricture to maintain a good flow of bile, much like stents are sometimes used in coronary arteries to maintain blood flow to the heart.

Medications can be used to treat the symptoms of PSC, such as itching. Unfortunately, there is no cure for PSC, and no medications are known to slow down the damage to the bile ducts. Even removal of the colon to treat ulcerative colitis or Crohn's colitis does not stop the progression of PSC.

75. How do Crohn's disease and ulcerative colitis cause you to become anemic?

Anemia is a condition that occurs when the body is depleted of red blood cells. The two main causes of anemia are loss of blood and decreased production of red blood cells. Blood loss is most commonly caused by gastrointestinal bleeding. Rapid gastrointestinal bleeding is uncommon in IBD and suggests that there is another potential source, such as a bleeding ulcer or bleeding from **diverticulosis**. Chronic, or slow, blood loss causing iron deficiency anemia is commonly seen in Crohn's disease and less commonly in ulcerative colitis. A variety of illnesses can cause anemia from decreased production of red blood cells, including iron and vitamin deficiencies, lead poisoning, bone marrow problems, chronic kidney failure, and certain blood disorders such as **sickle cell anemia** and **thalassemia**. Some medications may also cause anemia. Caveat: anyone over the age of 50 who develops new-onset iron deficiency anemia should be checked thoroughly for an underlying gastrointestinal cancer as a possible cause.

Individuals with Crohn's disease involving the small bowel can develop anemia for several reasons. To start with, inflammation or subsequent surgical removal of the small bowel can cause malabsorption that leads to inadequate uptake of vitamins and nutrients. Bodily stores of iron, vitamin B_{12}, and folate can become depleted, leading to anemia. Also, commonly used medications in Crohn's disease and ulcerative colitis such as azathioprine (Imuran) and methotrexate can also cause anemia; the anemia can sometimes be severe enough to warrant stopping the medication. Last, active Crohn's disease or ulcerative colitis can lead to anemia of chronic disease as a result of stress on the body as a whole.

Symptoms of chronic anemia include tiredness, pale skin, shortness of breath on exertion, and decreased exercise capacity. This happens because red blood cells deliver oxygen to the various tissues and organs of the body. As the number of red blood cells decreases in

Chronic, or slow, blood loss causing iron deficiency anemia is commonly seen in Crohn's disease and less commonly in ulcerative colitis.

Extraintestinal Manifestations

anemia, the body does not get enough oxygen to work at full capacity. If you have underlying heart disease, chest pain and shortness of breath can be important signals that your heart is under excessive stress and that the anemia needs to be corrected immediately with a blood transfusion. Severe anemia can lead to a rapid pulse, decrease in blood pressure, and episodes of passing out. When this occurs, an immediate blood transfusion is usually needed. However, the majority of IBD patients with chronic anemia do not need blood transfusions, but usually get better with folate, B$_{12}$, or iron supplementation. As mentioned in Question 45, bleeding from ulcerative colitis does not usually cause significant anemia and is rarely severe enough to require a blood transfusion.

76. Am I more likely to get a blood clot if I have IBD?

Individuals with Crohn's disease and ulcerative colitis have a higher risk for developing a blood clot, also called a **thrombosis**. These can occur anywhere in the body, but mostly in the legs. When the blood clot affects the superficial veins in the skin, it is called **thrombophlebitis**. When the blood clot affects the deeper veins, it is called a **deep venous thrombosis**, or **DVT**. Symptoms of a DVT include pain in the calf muscle, swelling, or redness. A DVT can break off from the veins in the legs and travel to the lungs where it can become lodged. This is called a **pulmonary embolus**, or **PE**. A person who has a PE may experience shortness of breath, increased heart rate, pain in the chest, or pain in the ribs or chest when taking a deep breath. Large or multiple PEs can be life-threatening. Blood clots can also occur in other blood

Individuals with Crohn's disease and ulcerative colitis have a higher risk for developing a blood clot, also called a thrombosis.

vessels, including those that supply blood to the liver and intestines. When this occurs, blood flow to the intestines can be lost, which is called **mesenteric ischemia**. Individuals who have an inherited disorder called **antiphospholipid antibody syndrome** are more prone to blood clots not only in the veins but also in the arteries, which can lead to potential complications such as stroke and miscarriage. Patients on home TPN (see Question 55) are also at risk for blood clots because they have an indwelling IV line in their vein that can become clogged with a blood clot.

Individuals who develop blood clots may need to be treated with blood-thinning medications. Most are initially hospitalized and given an IV infusion of heparin sodium or an injection with enoxaparin (Lovenox). For long-term treatment, oral warfarin sodium is given. All three drugs are blood-thinning medications that help prevent future blood clots from forming. If you have a single episode of blood clot formation, your doctor may decide that you need to take warfarin sodium for up to six months. Usually, you may undergo a variety of blood tests to detect any other underlying genetic disorders that can make you more prone to developing blood clots.

Warfarin sodium (coumadin) can be a challenging medication to take because every patient reacts to it differently and requires a different dose. Two blood tests, called the prothrombin time (**PT**) and the international normalized ratio (**INR**), are used to monitor warfarin sodium. These blood tests help to determine the level of thinness of the blood. Your physician will check the PT/INR frequently until an appropriate dose can be established. The PT/INR is then checked less frequently, but still on a regular basis. Other medications, especially antibiotics, can interact with coumadin; many of the foods we eat, such as green leafy vegetables can interact with coumadin as well. As you can imagine, these blood-thinning medications can leave patients vulnerable not only to easy bruising but also to more severe bleeding from things such as skin cuts and stomach ulcers. Individuals on warfarin sodium have to be careful not to get injured, especially with head trauma, because it can lead to massive bleeding and death. This medication should be taken only under the strict supervision of a doctor. If you have bloody diarrhea associated with an ulcerative colitis flare, warfarin sodium will not necessarily make it significantly worse because the bleeding of ulcerative colitis is usually superficial and looks worse than it actually is.

PART NINE

Sexuality, Reproductive Issues, and Pregnancy

Is it safe to have a baby if I have IBD?

Is there a best time to get pregnant if I have IBD?

Should I continue to take my IBD medications during pregnancy?

More ...

77. Is it safe to have a baby if I have IBD?

Yes, it is safe to have a baby if you have Crohn's disease or ulcerative colitis. IBD most commonly affects young men and women during their childbearing years, so naturally many individuals with IBD are concerned about whether they can safely have children. Being pregnant does not appear to pose any increased risk to women who have IBD as compared to those who do not have IBD. Nevertheless, studies have shown that women who have active, poorly controlled Crohn's disease or ulcerative colitis during pregnancy are more at risk for miscarriage, premature delivery, and stillbirth. While there are some suggestions in medical literature that even women in remission may have a very small risk for premature delivery and low birth weight, in general, women with Crohn's disease or ulcerative colitis who are in remission are at little, if any, increased risk for a pregnancy-related complication. It is important to note, however, that even for healthy women without Crohn's disease or ulcerative colitis, there is a 2–3% chance of having a complication during pregnancy. In other words, although it is safe to have a baby if you have Crohn's disease or ulcerative colitis in remission, there is still some degree of risk inherent in any pregnancy. When all is said and done, most women with Crohn's disease and ulcerative colitis have normal pregnancies and deliver healthy babies.

Yes, it is safe to have a baby if you have Crohn's disease or ulcerative colitis.

78. Is there a best time to get pregnant if I have IBD?

The best time to get pregnant is when your Crohn's disease or ulcerative colitis is in remission. Women in remission are at no greater risk for a pregnancy-related complication than the general population is. In addition, if a woman is in remission at the time of conception, she is likely to remain in remission for the duration of the pregnancy. However, if that same woman were to have active IBD symptoms at the time of conception, she would be likely to continue to have active symptoms for the remainder of the pregnancy. Therefore, strongly consider delaying pregnancy until your IBD has been brought under control.

The best time to get pregnant is when your Crohn's disease or ulcerative colitis is in remission.

A woman's overall health and fitness is also vital to having a normal pregnancy. The basic rules that apply to any pregnancy, such as not drinking or smoking, apply to pregnant women with Crohn's disease or ulcerative colitis. It is good advice to discuss with your gastroenterologist any plans for future pregnancies early on. He or she can help you plan ahead and make good decisions when the time comes. Along the same lines, you should choose an obstetrician who is experienced in caring for a mother with IBD. Crohn's disease and ulcerative colitis should not interfere with your hopes of having a family.

Jennifer's comment:

After 3 years of marriage and more than 5 years in remission, my husband and I decided that we were ready to start a family. However, we were concerned that getting pregnant would pose a significant risk to my health and the health of our unborn child. We also had a number of questions. Would pregnancy activate my Crohn's? How could my disease be treated if I were pregnant? Would our child be at risk for major birth defects or abnormalities caused by the various medications and surgeries I had been exposed to?

My husband and I knew that getting pregnant would require a great deal of methodical planning and careful timing given my history with Crohn's. As a result, discussing my intentions to get pregnant as well as my questions and concerns with my gastroenterologist was an important first step. My doctor assured me that my chances for a normal *pregnancy were no different than any other woman's without IBD. However, despite the fact I had been symptom free of Crohn's for more than 5 years, he urged me to undergo a colonoscopy to ensure my Crohn's was not active, which would influence which medications he would keep me on. My gynecologist concurred: a colonoscopy would provide her with critical baseline information that would be used to monitor my health throughout my pregnancy.*

My desire to have a pregnancy that was both safe for me and my unborn child outweighed my anxiety about the test and the results. Thankfully, we received the news we hoped for—I was still in remission and in perfect health to have a baby. Armed with this information, my husband and I happily set off to tackle the next big hurdle: getting pregnant.

79. Will having Crohn's disease or ulcerative colitis affect my ability to conceive?

Crohn's disease and ulcerative colitis in and of themselves should not affect your ability to conceive a child.

Crohn's disease and ulcerative colitis in and of themselves should not affect your ability to conceive a child. It is important to remember that up to 8–10% of healthy couples in the United States have difficulty conceiving, including those with Crohn's disease or ulcerative colitis. Some studies have shown that women with IBD tend to have fewer children in general, especially if Crohn's disease or ulcerative colitis is diagnosed before the first pregnancy. The reason for this is unclear. Fortunately, newer and better medications that are generally safe to continue during pregnancy can enable women with IBD to feel more secure about conceiving a healthy child.

Whereas having Crohn's disease or ulcerative colitis may not make it more difficult for you to conceive, having undergone surgery for IBD can. Any woman who has had lower abdominal or pelvic surgery for any reason, or who has had a pelvic infection, may have difficulty conceiving. This probably is a result of scar tissue formation interfering with the normal reproductive process. Unfortunately, individuals with Crohn's disease and ulcerative colitis may find themselves in just this situation. Starting when they are relatively young, IBD patients often need to undergo surgery and also can develop intra-abdominal and pelvic infections. Women with ulcerative colitis who have had ileal pouch surgery have markedly increased rates of infertility.

80. Why do I feel like I have no sex drive?

Active symptoms from Crohn's disease and ulcerative colitis, such as fatigue, abdominal pain, diarrhea, and perianal disease can make intercourse seem less appealing. An IBD flare can also place a good deal of stress on a relationship. Medications such as prednisone can cause emotional problems such as weepiness, depression, irritability, and insomnia. Weight gain from prednisone can also make patients feel less desirable. Active IBD can leave you feeling tired and stressed out, with sex being the last thing on your mind. Once your symptoms are better controlled, you can start to get back on track.

Active symptoms from Crohn's disease and ulcerative colitis, such as fatigue, abdominal pain, diarrhea, and perianal disease can make intercourse seem less appealing.

Some patients who have had surgery for IBD, especially those who have an ileostomy or colostomy, may feel less attractive or have a decreased libido as a result of struggles with body image. In addition, women with perianal disease or those who have had pouch surgery can experience painful intercourse.

Enlisting the help of friends, family, and IBD support groups can provide a needed emotional foothold when you deal with these tough issues. Also, talk openly with your spouse or partner. Finally, it is always a good idea to mention any loss of sexual drive to your physician—sometimes it may be because of a hormonal imbalance that can be corrected with appropriate therapy. Even if you have no hormonal imbalance, it is important for your physician to be aware of how IBD is affecting your overall well-being.

81. Can IBD affect fertility in men?

Crohn's disease and ulcerative colitis do not cause fertility problems in men. However, sulfasalazine, a drug commonly used to treat IBD, can cause decreased sperm count, reduced sperm motility, and abnormal sperm shape. This can happen in as many as 80% of men taking this medication. Fortunately, this side effect is quickly reversible within 2 months of stopping sulfasalazine. This effect on sperm has not been found with any of the other aminosalicylates (olsalazine, mesalamine, mesalamine CR, or balsalzide). Therefore, when a man on sulfasalazine would like to conceive a child, he should be switched to one of these other medications, which work just as effectively for Crohn's disease and ulcerative colitis.

Crohn's disease and ulcerative colitis do not cause fertility problems in men.

82. What is the effect of pregnancy on Crohn's disease and ulcerative colitis?

If a woman with Crohn's disease or ulcerative colitis is in remission at the time of conception, she will likely stay in remission for the duration of the pregnancy. On the other hand, if a woman's IBD is active at the time of conception, she is likely to continue to have symptoms throughout the pregnancy. For this reason, it is recommended that a woman should not become pregnant in the setting of active Crohn's disease or ulcerative colitis. A woman in remission at the start of her pregnancy who decides to stop her IBD medications is also at risk for a flare, just as she would be if she stopped her medications at any other time.

Women who have had an ileostomy or colostomy may rarely develop difficulties with their **ostomy** as a result of the enlarging uterus pushing aside the bowel. This should resolve on its own once the baby has been delivered.

83. Should I continue to take my IBD medications during pregnancy?

It is important for your health and the health of your baby that you continue taking your IBD medications during pregnancy. (Question 84 discusses which medications are safe to use.) In general, there is a greater risk to the baby in stopping your medications and potentially developing a flare during the pregnancy than any potential side effects from the medications. A flare during pregnancy, especially if surgery is required,

It is important for your health and the health of your baby that you continue taking your IBD medications during pregnancy.

is far more dangerous for your baby than any potential risks from IBD medications. Many women have reservations about taking *any* medications during pregnancy. The best approach is to be honest with your doctor about your feelings and have good communication about the risks and benefits of continuing medications to maintain the best control of your IBD. Doctors care as much about you and your family as you do and want the best for everyone involved. That is why the most important decisions about continuing medications during pregnancy can also be the hardest ones to make.

Jennifer's comment:

One of the most difficult decisions I was forced to make when planning for pregnancy was whether to continue to take my Crohn's medications. I had been taking mesalamine (Asacol) and 6-MP since my last surgery (for more than 5 years at this point) in an effort to prolong my remission. Although I was worried about the implications of stopping my medications altogether, I was unwilling to consider any medication that might pose even the smallest risk to my unborn child.

I spent a lot of time discussing my options with Dr. Warner as well as my gynecologist and my husband. Although Dr. Warner assured me that it was safe to continue taking mesalamine and 6-MP while pregnant, he took my concerns seriously and spent time discussing the trade-offs of stopping one or both of these medications. My husband and gynecologist had strong positions on the matter, but the decision was ultimately mine to make.

In the end, I made the decision to stop taking one of the two medications I was on. This decision was not made lightly, but in the end, it was the one I was most comfortable with.

Dr. Warner supported my decision, and together we discussed alternative treatment options in the event I might experience a recurrence of my Crohn's during pregnancy. We have also discussed a plan for putting me back on my medication once my baby is born.

My Crohn's medications alone did not ensure me good health during pregnancy; rather, my medications coupled with the open dialogue I have with Dr. Warner on these issues made the difference.

84. Are IBD medications safe to use during pregnancy?

The general consensus among IBD experts is that most medications used for the treatment of Crohn's disease and ulcerative colitis are safe during pregnancy (see Table 13). However, studies involving pregnant

The general consensus among IBD experts is that most medications used for the treatment of Crohn's disease and ulcerative colitis are safe during pregnancy.

Table 13 Crohn's Disease and Ulcerative Colitis Medications for Use During Pregnancy and Breastfeeding.

Medication	Category	Pregnancy	Breastfeeding
Aminosalicylates	B	Safe	Safe
Metronidazole	B	Safe	Probably safe
Infliximab	B	Safe	Safe
Corticosteroids	C	Safe	Safe
Ciprofloxacin	C	Safe	Not safe
Levofloxacin	C	Safe	Not safe
Azathioprine/6-MP	D	Probably safe	Not safe
Methotrexate	X	Not safe	Not safe
Thalidomide	X	Not safe	Not safe

women often are small and provide only limited information about the safety of drugs during pregnancy, as is true for all disorders and not just IBD. In most cases, physicians rely upon experience, and when it comes to the various medications used to treat Crohn's disease and ulcerative colitis, this means years of experience.

All medications have been categorized by the **FDA** regarding their risk in pregnancy (see Table 14). These guidelines are based mostly on studies involving animals and not necessarily humans. Almost all of the medications used in the treatment of IBD have been deemed safe to use during pregnancy (see Table 13).

The aminosalicylates (sulfasalazine, olsalazine, mesalamine, mesalamine CR, and balsalazide) are classified as category B and, therefore, are considered

Table 14   FDA Ranking System for Drug Safety During Pregnancy

Category A: Drugs that have been tested for safety in pregnancy and are found to be safe.

Category B: Drugs that have been extensively used during pregnancy and that do not appear to cause major birth defects or other problems.

Category C: Drugs that are more likely to cause a problem for the mother or the fetus; these drugs come with a warning that they should be used only if the benefits outweigh the risks.

Category D: Drugs that have clear health risks for the fetus.

Category X: Drugs that have been shown to cause birth defects and should never be taken during pregnancy.

safe to use during pregnancy. Women taking sulfasalazine should also take supplemental folic acid because of sulfasalazine's interference with this nutrient's absorption. (In fact, it is a good idea for all women hoping to become pregnant to supplement with folic acid to avoid birth defects, regardless of whether they have IBD.) Mesalamine enemas (Rowasa) and mesalamine suppositories (Canasa) are topical aminosalicylates and are also classified as category B.

Prednisone and budesonide are classified as category C and are commonly used during pregnancy. Prednisone, especially, is used in a wide variety of medical conditions. Azathioprine and 6-mercaptopurine (6-MP) have been listed as FDA category D because studies on pregnant animals showed harm to the fetus. However, exceedingly high doses were used on these animals, much higher than standard doses used in treating Crohn's disease and ulcerative colitis. We know from decades of experience with IBD as well as transplant patients who have become pregnant that these medications appear to be safe in humans. The antibiotics ciprofloxacin and levofloxacin, category C, and metronidazole, category B, are also likely to be safe for use during pregnancy. Infliximab is one of the newest medications and is classified as category B. A large and continuously growing database of patients has demonstrated that pregnant women taking Remicade do not appear to have increased risk of harm to the fetus compared to the general population.

Cyclosporine, classified as category C, is considered safe, but its use during pregnancy is more complicated than is the use of other medications. Cyclosporine is often used in patients who are hospitalized with a severe ulcerative colitis flare and who are not getting better with intravenous corticosteroids. As you can imagine, these patients are very sick and may need surgery if they don't improve. Surgery for IBD during pregnancy can cause risk to the fetus and should be performed only as a last resort. Cyclosporine is used as an alternative to surgery and has an 80% likelihood of successfully treating the colitis and inducing a remission. However, cyclosporine's side effects can be severe, including anaphylactic shock, elevated blood pressure, and seizures, and poses a significant risk to the fetus. As always, the bottom line is to avoid these situations altogether by getting IBD under control before pregnancy.

85. Are there any Crohn's disease and ulcerative colitis medications that are not safe during pregnancy?

The two IBD medications that are not considered safe and should absolutely be avoided during pregnancy are methotrexate and thalidomide (category X). Unlike other medications for Crohn's disease and ulcerative colitis, these have been shown to increase the risk of birth defects in babies. Women who are sexually active and are taking these medications must use a medically accepted method of birth control. Both men and women should wait at least 3 months after stopping methotrexate and thalidomide before considering pregnancy. In addition, any woman who is taking one of these medications and would like to get pregnant should also switch to a safer medication prior to attempting to conceive to avoid having a flare during pregnancy.

The two IBD medications that are not considered safe and should absolutely be avoided during pregnancy are methotrexate and thalidomide (category X).

86. Can I take IBD medications while I am breastfeeding?

Many of the medications listed as safe during pregnancy are also considered safe for use during breastfeeding. Medications that are not recommended for breast feeding mothers include ciprofloxacin, levofloxacin, azathioprine (Imuran), and 6-MP. However, the risks to the mother of stopping azathioprine and 6-MP and potentially experiencing a flare need to be carefully weighed against the benefits of breastfeeding. It is important to remember that if you have a flare, you may be too ill to breastfeed and may need to begin taking additional medication that also may not be safe for use during breastfeeding. So, although you may prefer to breastfeed and should be allowed to if you can, bottle-feeding may be the safest option if the alternative is an IBD flare in a new mother.

Many medications listed as safe during pregnancy are also considered safe for use during breastfeeding.

87. Can I still have a vaginal delivery if I have perianal Crohn's disease, or do I need to have a C-section?

Women with Crohn's disease who have had perianal disease (abscess, fistula, or fissure) need to avoid an **episiotomy** because of the risk that the incision may not properly heal. Delivery by caesarean section (C-section) is usually recommended. This needs to be judged on a case-by-case basis depending upon the severity of the perianal disease and whether it is active or has been dormant for many years. Some cases of perianal disease occur for the first time ever following an episiotomy and the trauma of childbirth. However, these situations are unusual and should not necessarily influence your final decision.

88. Which tests or X rays for Crohn's disease and ulcerative colitis are safe during pregnancy?

Radiation exposure during pregnancy is a common concern. X rays use a type of ionized radiation that can potentially harm a fetus and should be avoided by all women during pregnancy. Even though the doses of ionized radiation during routine X rays are too low to pose harm to adults, radiation can affect the developing fetus and cause intrauterine death, malformation, disturbances to growth and development, and birth defects. The risks are highest in the first trimester when the fetal organs are still forming. (That's why whenever you have an X ray, the technician asks whether you are pregnant or think that you could be pregnant.) Nevertheless, if a pregnant woman is having a medical emergency and an X ray is needed to make the diagnosis, it may be unavoidable. Technicians can modify the X ray itself and shield the uterus with a lead apron to minimize radiation exposure to the fetus.

The types of imaging studies that involve potentially harmful ionized radiation include abdominal and chest X rays, CT scans, upper GI series with small bowel follow-through, barium enema, and **angiography** (a specialized test used to look at blood vessels). These tests should also be avoided if possible during pregnancy. Again, this recommendation changes in an emergency situation. The imminent risks to the mother's health need to be weighed against the potential risks to the fetus. Doctors and patients usually decide together in times like these, taking into account how badly the test is needed.

Ultrasound does not use radiation and is safe for use in pregnancy. The type of ultrasound used to look at abdominal organs is the same as the type of ultrasound used to monitor the growing fetus in a pregnant woman.

MRI scans use nonionized radiation, which is different from the potentially harmful ionized radiation used in X rays and related tests mentioned earlier. MRI scans are probably safe during pregnancy, but not enough information is known to be completely sure. Studies to date have shown no ill effects to the fetus with MRI scans. Gadolinium, the contrast sometimes used in an MRI scan, may potentially pose a small risk of harm to the fetus; it should be avoided during pregnancy.

Upper endoscopy, colonoscopy, and sigmoidoscopy have been deemed safe during pregnancy, but should be performed only if there is a strong indication to do so and not as routine tests. Endoscopy can provide a safer alternative to radiologic or surgical procedures during pregnancy. Some of the intravenous medications used for sedation during endoscopy are safer to use during pregnancy than others are. If you need an endoscopic procedure during pregnancy, your gastroenterologist will choose medications least harmful to the fetus.

ERCP is an advanced endoscopic procedure used to treat various complications of gallstone disease and illnesses such as primary sclerosing cholangitis of the liver (see Question 74). An ERCP may be used in a pregnant woman with active gallstone disease as an alternative to surgery. ERCP should be used only if absolutely necessary because it usually involves ionized radiation exposure from X rays. As with other imaging tests, the doctors and nurses performing the ERCP will take special care to limit radiation exposure to the fetus.

89. Can I safely have surgery for Crohn's disease or ulcerative colitis during pregnancy?

Routine surgery should be avoided during pregnancy because it poses a significant risk of harm to the fetus.

Routine surgery should be avoided during pregnancy because it poses a significant risk of harm to the fetus. In an emergency situation, however, surgery may become necessary to save the life of the mother and, therefore, the fetus. As mentioned earlier, whenever an emergency arises, you and your doctors need to discuss it carefully to assess the risks and benefits of surgery to both you and your fetus. In the case of Crohn's disease or ulcerative colitis, doctors usually have exhausted all medical options before considering surgery. If a pregnant woman is sick enough to require emergency surgery, chances are that the medications have either failed to work or the doctors think it is too risky to wait until the medications become effective. If surgery absolutely must be performed during pregnancy, the optimal time is during the second trimester because the anesthetics used during surgery will have the least effect on the growing fetus. Also, in the second trimester, the uterus is not yet large enough to distort the position of other organs within the abdomen.

90. Will prior surgery for Crohn's disease or ulcerative colitis affect my pregnancy or delivery?

Women with active anal disease, such as fistulas or abscesses, or recent anal disease are usually recommended to undergo an elective caesarean section to avoid the potential for any further damage to the anus and rectum that can ensue during a vaginal delivery. This is because even in the most routine vaginal delivery, the mother may have a vaginal tear or require an episiotomy. In the setting of active Crohn's disease involving the anus and surrounding region, a vaginal tear or episiotomy may not heal properly, which could potentially result in permanent damage to the anus and lead to fecal incontinence. Women who have a history of anal or perianal disease from many years earlier may be able to have a safe vaginal delivery. However, because risk of damage to the anus still exists, you and your obstetrician should carefully consider an elective caesarian section. If you and your obstetrician decide on a vaginal delivery and an episiotomy becomes necessary, the incision should be made away from the site of prior anal disease. An obstetrician may also opt to perform a caesarian section in the setting of an ileoanal pouch to avoid potentially damaging the pouch. However, many women with an ileal pouch have had successful vaginal deliveries; having an ileal pouch is not considered a contraindication to a normal, vaginal delivery.

A prior intestinal resection should not have any effect on pregnancy and delivery. However, women with an ileostomy or colostomy are at a slightly increased risk for a **prolapsed ostomy** (which is when the ostomy protrudes, or sticks out, more than usual) and for a bowel obstruction. This is because of the mechanical effect of the enlarged uterus displacing the intestines.

Finally, it is normal for a woman who is pregnant to develop altered bowel habits. This is more pronounced in a pregnant woman with an ileal pouch, who often notices an increased frequency of stools; this resolves after delivery.

91. Will Crohn's disease and ulcerative colitis affect my periods? Can they make PMS worse?

Evidence suggests that women with Crohn's disease or ulcerative colitis are likely to experience menstrual irregularities.

Evidence suggests that women with Crohn's disease or ulcerative colitis are likely to experience menstrual irregularities. This effect on the menstrual cycle is most pronounced if you have a severe IBD flare and lose a good deal of weight, in which case your periods may become irregular or may stop altogether. However, these effects are not unique to IBD and can happen in many different situations—a significant medical illness, months of daily vigorous exercise, or as a result of eating disorders, such as anorexia nervosa, for example. For a woman with IBD, the menstrual cycle is likely to return to normal once the flare has been brought under control.

In addition to the effect that Crohn's disease or ulcerative colitis can have on menstruation, menstruation in turn can affect your Crohn's disease or ulcerative colitis. IBD symptoms may worsen just before your period and may improve at the end of menstruation. The reason for this is unclear, although many healthy women report having a degree of nausea and constipation just before their periods and a change to loose stools once their period starts.

Crohn's disease and ulcerative colitis do not appear to have any effect on premenstrual syndrome (**PMS**) symptoms; however, if you are prone to mood swings just before your period, medications such as prednisone can make your mood swings worse, so be prepared.

92. If I have Crohn's disease or ulcerative colitis, what is the chance that my children will have it? Should my family members be tested?

If you have Crohn's disease or ulcerative colitis, there is about a 4–9% chance that you will have a child with IBD. If both parents have Crohn's disease or ulcerative colitis, the risk for the child increases to 36%. However, as mentioned in Question 9, this risk is small, and just because you have IBD doesn't automatically mean that your kids will have it, too.

Several genes have been identified as associated with Crohn's disease and ulcerative colitis. One is called the *NOD2/CARD 15* gene, which has more than 60 variations. For example, three of these *NOD2/CARD 15* gene variations have been identified in 27% of people with Crohn's disease specifically involving the ileum. It is important to remember, though, that although these genes are involved in Crohn's disease and ulcerative

If you have Crohn's disease or ulcerative colitis, there is about a 4–9% chance that you will have a child with IBD. If both parents have Crohn's disease or ulcerative colitis, the risk for the child increases to 36%.

colitis, they are only part of the story. The *NOD2/ CARD 15* gene is believed to play the role of a permissive gene, meaning that the gene cannot cause IBD by itself, but can help facilitate the expression of Crohn's disease or ulcerative colitis. In other words, even if you carry one of these genes, you will not automatically develop Crohn's disease or ulcerative colitis. Rather, Crohn's disease or ulcerative colitis may be caused by a combination of genetic influences and an environmental trigger, such as a bacterium.

Genetic testing is not widely available at this time, nor is it currently recommended for families and children of individuals with IBD. Regardless, scientific research about the genetics of IBD is a growing and exciting field. By examining the underlying genetics of IBD, physicians may be better able to understand and predict different patterns and degrees of severity in Crohn's disease and ulcerative colitis.

PART TEN

Lifestyle

Does stress affect Crohn's disease and
ulcerative colitis?

Can changing my lifestyle help with my IBD?

Can I drink alcohol if I have IBD?

More ...

93. Does stress affect Crohn's disease and ulcerative colitis?

There is *no* scientific evidence to support any of the following statements:

1. Emotional stress can cause a person to develop Crohn's disease or ulcerative colitis.
2. Emotional stress can induce a flare of Crohn's disease or ulcerative colitis.
3. There is a higher incidence of major psychiatric illness in patients with Crohn's disease or ulcerative colitis than the general population.

What is known, however, is that patients with IBD, or any chronic illness, who concomitantly suffer from depression have a more difficult clinical course than a chronically ill patient without depression. In other words, depressed people may not deal as well with illness than people without depression do. In addition, some of the medications that are used to treat Crohn's disease and ulcerative colitis, most notably prednisone, may cause severe mood swings, tremulousness, insomnia, depression, and, rarely, homicidal thoughts.

This is not to say that an individual under stress will never have gastrointestinal symptoms such as nausea, vomiting, cramps, bloating, and/or diarrhea. In fact, it is exceedingly common for someone under emotional stress to have just these types of symptoms—but they are not from active Crohn's disease or ulcerative colitis; these symptoms are a normal functional reaction in individuals under stress.

Lifestyle

Ken's comment:

I can't say that times of stress have caused my ulcerative colitis to flare. Instead, stressful times result in general intestinal discomfort, as well as irritability, headaches, and a short temper. The point is although stress doesn't necessarily make my ulcerative colitis worse, it makes me feel worse, and that can manifest in ways that aren't helped by the fact that I have ulcerative colitis.

The solution? Look for ways to relieve stress. Exercise is a great outlet. Reading to my kids, listening to music, and going for long walks are all ways to reduce the stress and maintain some semblance of well-being.

Jennifer's comment:

Type A personality. Overachiever. Perfectionist. These are some of the words and phrases that my friends and family (and just about anyone who has met me) commonly use to describe me. And in all my years of living with Crohn's, the list of characteristics attributed to me has never changed. This is who I am.

Given these inherent traits, one of the most frustrating aspects of living with Crohn's disease over the years has been listening to friends and family tell me that I brought this disease on myself by being "too stressed" or "too busy." I heard this when I was first diagnosed with Crohn's as a high school honors student preparing for college and involved in a dozen extracurricular activities. I heard it again after my first surgery and was warned to "take it easy" as I headed off to college. These comments resurfaced in full force when my Crohn's reappeared 4 years later while I was busy climbing the corporate ladder and living the fast-paced life of a twenty-something in New York City.

It would have been very easy to accept what all those people who love and care about me told me about my disease. But then I would have been forced to lead a different life (one without the excitement I thrive on) and give up on many of my hopes and dreams. Whereas I was willing to accept Crohn's disease as part of my life, I was not willing to accept anything less than the life I had planned for myself.

Over the years, my doctors have assured me that stress is not a trigger for this disease. Although I am in no way immune from the side effects of stress—it can aggravate my gastrointestinal tract even when I'm in remission—I know it is not the reason I have Crohn's. With my doctors' help, I have found a way to manage my disease while achieving amazing accomplishments in both my professional and personal life, which now include juggling life as a corporate executive, a wife, and an expectant mother.

Unfortunately, no amount of scientific evidence (or lack thereof) has been able to convince my friends and family that stress is not linked to my Crohn's. Over the years I have learned to accept their comments as expressions of love and concern rather than an admonition about the life I lead. I can only imagine how frustrating it is for them not to be able to find a solution to a disease that has the potential to cause me such pain. For them, a slow-paced, less stressful life has always been the solution. For me, it would be no life at all.

Lifestyle changes can often help to improve intestinal symptoms of Crohn's disease and ulcerative colitis.

94. Can changing my lifestyle help with my IBD?

Lifestyle changes can often help to improve intestinal symptoms of Crohn's disease and ulcerative colitis. As mentioned earlier, even in individuals who do not have

IBD can experience cramps, urgency, and diarrhea as a result of stress. Therefore, stress reduction often does lead to improvement in many of the symptoms associated with Crohn's disease and ulcerative colitis. Along the same lines, avoiding overeating, fatty and fried foods, and caffeine is also beneficial. And although it may be old-fashioned, getting a good night's sleep and resting when you are fatigued are helpful as well. However, although these lifestyle changes can provide symptomatic relief from IBD, they won't completely heal or cure the underlying disease. For this reason, even if a change in lifestyle does make you feel better, you should not stop prescription medications before speaking with your physician. Regardless, lifestyle changes go a long way in improving your overall quality of life with respect to your IBD.

Ken's comment:

Findings ways to eliminate stress, negativity, or unpleasant situations through lifestyle changes are bigger than just ways to manage IBD. For me, my overall health and well-being are directly related to my ability to maintain a positive outlook, gain fulfillment from my job, and generally be happy and optimistic. I wouldn't advocate a lifestyle change just to help with IBD; instead, change your lifestyle to improve your life!

Take time out for yourself. All work and no play does not make for a well-rounded individual, and likewise, dwelling on the fact that you have IBD and taking on a negative attitude aren't very enjoyable. I work in a job that requires a lot of travel, and that alone can be stressful and unpleasant. So, when I'm away, I make sure I can maintain balance—by taking a few extra days and having my family join me at a nice location, by sneaking out for a baseball game when I'm in a new city, or by making sure I keep up with my exercise routine when I'm away from home. To be sure, none of these activities is a direct way to alleviate IBD symptoms, but they are all ways to keep a positive outlook, decompress, and make the daily struggles—including managing my ulcerative colitis—a little easier.

Jennifer's comments:

I've discovered that certain lifestyle changes can help me more effectively manage my Crohn's disease.

Over the years, I have found that eliminating certain foods from my diet (especially greasy, fried, fatty foods) and ensuring I get 8 hours of sleep a night have gone a long way in improving how I feel, especially when my Crohn's is active. Regular exercise (power walking either outside or on a treadmill is what works for me) has also proved very helpful.

There are certainly some things I'd rather not live without even though my body tells me I should—like my morning cup (or three) of coffee and afternoon Diet Coke. I'm just willing to live with the consequences of these indulgences.

95. I know smoking is bad for me, but I've heard that smoking can actually make IBD better—is this true?

It has long been known that a connection between cigarette smoking and IBD exists.

It has long been known that a connection between cigarette smoking and IBD exists. Ulcerative colitis often appears within a year or 2 after someone quits smoking. If that same person has a flare, smoking cigarettes has a positive effect and improves the ulcerative colitis symptoms. Using a nicotine patch can have a similar beneficial effect on controlling active ulcerative colitis symptoms. Nicotine's side effects including headache, light-headedness, and nausea as well as the inability of a nicotine patch to maintain a long-term remission limit its use. In addition, smoking cigarettes is hazardous to your health and therefore should not be used as a treatment for ulcerative colitis. In Crohn's disease, on the other hand, smoking cigarette smoking has a deleterious effect. Crohn's disease patients who smoke are more likely to have difficult-to-control symptoms, require more aggressive drug therapy, and have a recurrence of Crohn's disease after surgery. Second-hand smoke has similar effects.

96. Do I have to take any precautions if I want to exercise?

Regular exercise, along with eating a healthy diet, helps promote a long and healthy life. Patients with Crohn's disease and ulcerative colitis are encouraged to engage in routine exercise, taking a few precautions first. Individuals with IBD who are in the middle of a flare and feel fatigued and worn out should never push themselves to work out, which only leads them to feel even more run down and take longer to fully recover from the flare. In other words, although regular exercise is beneficial in the long term, at times it can do more harm than good in the short term. So, exercise to stay fit, but only if you are fit enough to exercise.

Regular exercise, along with eating a healthy diet, helps promote a long and healthy life.

Crohn's disease and ulcerative colitis patients also have to be extra careful not to become dehydrated. Individuals with IBD often limit liquid intake to avoid having diarrhea, sometimes even to the point of becoming borderline dehydrated. Add to this the additional bodily fluid losses that normally result from exercising, and dehydration becomes a real risk. In these individuals, a careful balance needs to be maintained between taking in enough fluid to prevent dehydration, but not so much as to lead to diarrhea. Glucose and electrolyte-based solutions, such as Gatorade and Crystal Light, are products that are more likely to help maintain this balance, whereas plain water, especially ice-cold water, may not be as well absorbed and could potentially cause cramps and diarrhea.

Finally, patients with Crohn's disease or ulcerative colitis who have undergone surgery run a small chance of developing an incisional hernia, which is a hernia at the site of the surgical incision. These patients feel a small bulge at the incisional site that gets bigger when bearing down, such as when lifting a heavy object or doing sit-ups, and then becomes smaller after the abdomen has become more relaxed. Incisional hernias are not specific to IBD patients or IBD surgery and can develop after any type of operation. Anyone with a hernia should avoid exercises that cause the hernia to pop out, such as sit-ups, abdominal crunches, and weightlifting, because the hernia can become stuck out and may not go back in. This is called an incarcerated hernia and requires an operation to be repaired.

There is no inherent reason why an individual with Crohn's disease or ulcerative colitis cannot drink alcohol.

97. Can I drink alcohol if I have IBD?

There is no inherent reason why an individual with Crohn's disease or ulcerative colitis cannot drink alcohol. Alcohol has never been shown to induce an IBD flare or make IBD more difficult to treat. While alcohol can cause GI upset with cramps and diarrhea, and heavy alcohol use is known to cause alcoholic gastritis, these are direct effects of the alcohol on the gastrointestinal tract and are not related to the presence of

IBD. So while some patients with IBD report that consuming alcohol makes their symptoms worse, it is probably from alcohol-induced GI upset, and not from alcohol directly affecting their Crohn's disease or ulcerative colitis. As is generally recommended, alcohol should be consumed only in moderation and never to excess.

It is generally considered safe to drink limited amounts of alcohol while you are taking most medications used to treat Crohn's disease and ulcerative colitis. One strict exception is metronidazole—patients taking metronidazole should never drink alcohol, even in small quantities, because the combination of metronidazole and alcohol leads to severe stomach upset with uncontrollable nausea and vomiting. This is known as an Antabuse effect. Disulfiram (Antabuse) is a drug prescribed for alcoholics to make them want to stop drinking because it creates these severe gastrointestinal side effects whenever they drink alcohol while taking this drug.

Lifestyle

PART ELEVEN

IBD in Children and the Elderly

Does IBD occur in children? How is it different than in adults?

Can IBD occur in the elderly?

More . . .

98. Does IBD occur in children? How is it different than in adults?

Peak incidence of Crohn's disease and ulcerative colitis occurs in people between the ages of 15 and 25 years. However, Crohn's disease and ulcerative colitis have been diagnosed in very young children and, in rare instances, infants. Most are diagnosed in late childhood or early adolescence. Both children and adults who suffer from Crohn's disease or ulcerative colitis can have similar symptoms, but children are at risk for unique complications, including growth problems and delayed onset of puberty. Children with Crohn's disease or ulcerative colitis also can have very different symptoms from adults. They may develop more non-bowel symptoms, such as skin rashes, joint problems, fevers, and generalized feelings of sickness. They may not eat as well as other children or lag behind others in height and weight. This predominance of nonbowel symptoms can often make Crohn's disease and ulcerative colitis harder to detect and diagnose in children. The treatments for Crohn's disease and ulcerative colitis can also affect children differently. Specifically, prednisone may lead to growth problems in children.

Pediatric gastroenterologists are specially trained to treat Crohn's disease and ulcerative colitis in children. As part of their evaluation, children may require an upper endoscopy or colonoscopy and it is normal for them to be more anxious or fearful about these procedures than adults. In these situations, **general anesthesia**, which provides for deep sedation, is often used during these procedures, in contrast to adults, who usually require only moderate sedation.

Peak incidence of Crohn's disease and ulcerative colitis occurs in people between the ages of 15 and 25 years.

Although Crohn's disease and ulcerative colitis can occur in young children before the onset of puberty, it is much more common for IBD to first develop in the late teens. As mentioned earlier, even if you as a mother or father have Crohn's disease or ulcerative colitis, the chance of your child developing this disease is still very small. Although you cannot help but worry about this, you should try to refrain from reading too much into the usual colds and tummy aches that kids get in the natural course of growing up.

99. Can IBD occur in the elderly?

Although Crohn's disease and ulcerative colitis most commonly initially present between the ages of 15 and 40 years, people of any age can develop Crohn's disease or ulcerative colitis. However, the elderly may react differently to the onset of IBD, as well as any illness, from those who are younger. Whereas younger persons usually are able to verbalize specifically that they have abdominal pain and diarrhea, an elderly person with these symptoms may only become confused or withdrawn, stop eating, sleep too much, or develop incontinence. Because other illnesses may mimic IBD, physicians may need to do additional testing to make sure that an elderly person does not have another disorder that looks similar to Crohn's disease or ulcerative colitis. At the same time, sometimes physicians neglect to consider a diagnosis of Crohn's disease or ulcerative colitis in the elderly because it is so much less common in this age group. For example, a very pleasant elderly woman suffered from persistent diarrhea for months while her doctors assumed that she was having recurring infections from "something she must have picked up from the nursing home." She was treated with multiple antibiotics, but her condition didn't seem to improve. A colonoscopy was finally performed, and the woman was found to have ulcerative colitis.

One type of bowel disease more common in the elderly that, to the untrained eye, can appear like Crohn's disease or ulcerative colitis is called colonic ischemia. This is a type of colitis that occurs when a temporary lack of proper blood flow to the colon occurs. Risk factors include vigorous exercise, significant drop in blood pressure, severe dehydration, and certain medications such as estrogens and blood pressure-lowering drugs. Colonic ischemia can cause symptoms of crampy abdominal pain with bloody diarrhea and can even look similar to Crohn's colitis or ulcerative colitis by colonoscopy. However, colonic ischemia can usually be differentiated from IBD by the patients' clinical presentation. Colonic ischemia usually develops abruptly in a person who previously did not have any intestinal symptoms, whereas individuals with Crohn's disease or ulcerative colitis usually have had some prior intestinal symptoms. Colonic ischemia is treated with resting the bowel by not eating, with intravenous fluids, and by removal of offending medications. Another type of bowel disease that may mimic IBD is colon cancer. This should always be ruled out first before settling on a diagnosis of Crohn's disease or ulcerative colitis. Diverticulitis can also have a similar appearance to Crohn's disease.

Elderly individuals with Crohn's disease or ulcerative colitis are more prone to complications from medications used to treat their disease. Corticosteroids can be particularly troublesome in the elderly, especially in the setting of preexisting diabetes, cataracts, and osteoporosis. Compromising the immune system with medications such as azathioprine (Imuran) can lead to serious side effects such as pneumonia, which are harder for elderly people to fight. Because side effects can be more pronounced and cause greater consequences in the elderly, this population needs to be monitored much more closely by their physicians. Depending on the severity of an elderly person's Crohn's disease or ulcerative colitis, the individual may need to discuss with his or her doctor and family the risks and benefits of each medication in the face of potentially creating even bigger problems.

Elderly individuals with Crohn's disease or ulcerative colitis are more prone to complications from medications used to treat their disease.

IBD in Children and the Elderly

PART TWELVE

The Future of Crohn's Disease and Ulcerative Colitis

What does the future hold for the diagnosis and treatment of Crohn's disease and ulcerative colitis?

More ...

100. What does the future hold for the diagnosis and treatment of Crohn's disease and ulcerative colitis?

The past 10 to 15 years have witnessed great strides in understanding the basic **immunology** of IBD and dramatic advances in the treatment of IBD. With this strong foundation to grow upon, the future for individuals with IBD is both bright and hopeful. Two trends are likely to emerge in the coming years: delineation of the genetic basis for IBD and targeted immune-modulating therapy.

*The past 10 to 15 years have witnessed great strides in understanding the basic **immunology** of IBD and dramatic advances in the treatment of IBD. With this strong foundation to grow upon, the future for individuals with IBD is both bright and hopeful.*

The genetic basis for IBD is a complex subject that is still in its infancy. Active research is allowing physicians to gain insight into the genetic patterns that underlie IBD. Much like ocean currents that naturally landscape the coastlines, genetic patterns determine the landscape of IBD—whether you get Crohn's disease or ulcerative colitis, whether your symptoms are mild or severe, whether you respond to medical therapy, and whether you go into remission or need surgery. The knowledge about IBD that emerges from this research is expected to yield innovative drug therapy that will be able more closely to target the cells, proteins, and agents that cause Crohn's disease and ulcerative colitis.

Appendix

Lahey Clinic
Department of Gastroenterology
41 Mall Road
Burlington, MA 01805
Phone: 781-744-5100
Web site: www.lahey.org

American College of Gastroenterology
Web site: www.acg.gi.org

American Gastroenterological Association
Web site: www.gastro.org

American Liver Foundation
Web site: www.liverfoundation.org

Crohn's and Colitis Foundation of America
Web site: www.ccfa.org

Glossary

Abdominal cavity: The part of the body below the chest and above the pelvic bone that contains the internal organs, including the small intestine, colon, stomach, liver, pancreas, kidneys, and bladder.

Abdominal X ray: A radiologic examination that provides an image of structures and organs in the abdomen—helpful in detecting a bowel obstruction or perforation.

Abscess: A walled-off collection of pus; in Crohn's disease, an abscess is most commonly found around the anus or rectum, but can occur anywhere in the body.

Adhesion: Scar tissue that forms internally, usually after an operation; a common cause of bowel obstruction.

Adjunctive therapy: Using a drug or therapy in addition to the primary therapy.

Adrenal crisis: A sudden drop in blood pressure that occurs if a corticosteroid, such as prednisone, is abruptly discontinued.

Adverse effect: Side effect to a medication or treatment.

Aminosalicylate: A class of drugs used in Crohn's disease and ulcerative colitis.

Anastomosis: A surgically made connection between two structures in the body; in IBD, this is usually between two segments of intestine after a resection, or between the intestine and the skin to create an ileostomy or colostomy.

Anastomotic leak: Breakdown of the anastomosis, usually caused by an infection, in which intestinal bacteria leak out and cause an even worse infection.

Anemia: A lower-than-normal level of blood.

Angiography: A radiologic test that looks at the blood vessels.

Anorexia: An eating disorder in which someone does not want to eat.

Anoscopy: A procedure in which a rigid, short, straight, lighted tube is used to examine the anal canal; usually performed on a special tilt table that positions the patient with the head down and buttocks up. An excellent test to examine for an anal fissure or hemorrhoids.

Antibodies to infliximab (ATIs): Because infliximab (Remicade) is part mouse, the immune system detects that infliximab is foreign and creates these antibodies to fight against it.

Antimotility drugs: Class of drugs that slow down gastrointestinal motility; used to treat diarrhea.

Antineutrophil cytoplasmic antibody (ANCA): An antibody found in the blood that is associated with the presence of ulcerative colitis.

Antiphospholipid antibody syndrome: An inherited disorder that causes individuals to be more prone to form blood clots.

Anti-Saccharomyces cerevisiae antibody (ASCA): An antibody found in the blood that is associated with the presence of Crohn's disease.

Antispasmodic drugs: Class of drugs used to relieve painful bowel spasm.

Anus: The outside opening of the rectum.

Aphthous ulcers: Small ulcers that can occur in IBD.

Arthralgias: Joint soreness and stiffness.

Arthritis: Inflammation of the joints; individuals with arthritis often have pain, redness, tenderness, and swelling in the affected joints.

Atrophy: A slow deterioration, or thinning, of tissue.

Autoimmune: An inflammatory process in which your immune system attacks part of your own body, such as the colon in ulcerative colitis.

Bacterial overgrowth: A condition in which an overgrowth of normal intestinal flora occurs; usually seen in the setting of an intestinal stricture.

Barium enema: A radiologic examination of the rectum and colon performed by instilling barium through the rectum and taking X rays as it travels through the colon; an excellent test to detect strictures, inflammation, and fistulas in the colon.

Benign: A noncancerous growth.

Bile acids: Digestive enzymes synthesized in the liver and absorbed in the ileum; individuals with ileal disease or ileal resection are unable to absorb bile acids, which then enter the colon where they act as an irritant that causes diarrhea.

Bile duct: A channel through which bile flows from the liver to the intestines.

Biliary colic: Intense gallbladder pain caused by spasm.

Biopsy: Usually performed during an endoscopy, a small piece of mucosa (inside lining of the intestine) is removed and examined under a microscope; an excellent test to characterize types of inflammation and detect dysplasia and cancer.

Bisphosphonate: A class of drugs used to treat osteoporosis.

Bowel: Another name for intestine; that is, *small intestine* means the same as *small bowel.*

Bulimia: An eating disorder in which someone induces vomiting after eating, sometimes after eating large amounts of food, which is termed *binging* and *purging.*

Bypass operation: An operation in which a segment of diseased intestine is bypassed by connecting the healthy intestine above the diseased segment to the healthy intestine below.

Cancer: An uncontrolled growth of cells in the body that can form a tumor and can spread, or metastasize, to other areas of the body.

Capsule endoscopy: A test in which the patient swallows a large pill containing a camera and wears a sensor device on the abdomen; the capsule passes naturally through the small intestine while transmitting video images to the sensor, which stores data that can be downloaded to a computer.

Cataracts: A clouding of the eyes' natural lens; occurs naturally with age, but their development can be accelerated with chronic use of corticosteroids.

CCFA: Crohn's and Colitis Foundation of America

Celiac sprue: A malabsorption disorder characterized by intolerance to gluten, which is a protein found in wheat, barley, rye, and sometimes oats.

Cell: The smallest unit in the body; millions of cells attached together make up the organs and tissues.

Cholangiocarcinoma: Cancer of the bile ducts; can occur in primary sclerosing cholangitis (PSC).

Cholangiogram: X ray of the bile ducts; performed during an endoscopic procedure called an ERCP or by an MRI of the bile ducts.

Cholangitis: Infection of the bile ducts; can occur in primary sclerosing cholangitis (PSC).

Cholecystitis: Infection or inflammation of the gallbladder.

Cirrhosis: A condition in which the liver has become severely scarred; most commonly caused by excess alcohol use or viral infection, but can also be a result of medication.

Clostridium difficile (C. diff.): An unhealthy bacterium that can overpopulate the colon, usually as a result of antibiotic use, which leads to colitis symptoms that include diarrhea and cramps. It is treated by the antibiotics metronidazole (Flagyl) or vancomycin.

Colectomy: Surgical removal of the colon.

Colitis: Inflammation of the colon; can be a result of Crohn's disease, ulcerative colitis, or other diseases.

Colonic ischemia: Colon inflammation caused by lack of blood flow; also called ischemic colitis.

Colonic transit time: The time it takes for stool to travel from the beginning of the colon (the cecum) to the rectum.

Colonoscopy: An endoscopic procedure in which a small, thin, flexible lighted tube with a camera on the end is passed through the rectum into the colon and, at times, into the ileum; an excellent test to detect inflammation and strictures in the rectum, colon, and ileum, and one that allows for a biopsy to be taken.

Colostomy: Surgically created connection between the colon and skin to allow for the diversion of fecal material; the waste empties into a bag attached to the skin.

Corticosteroid: A potent anti-inflammatory drug.

Crohn's disease: An intestinal disease characterized by chronic intestinal inflammation; can affect any area of the gastrointestinal tract

Crohn's colitis: Crohn's disease of the colon

CT scan: Computed tomography scan; a radiologic test that uses X rays to create a detailed look inside the body; it is especially helpful in detecting abscesses and also useful in evaluating for bowel obstructions and perforation.

DALM: Dysplasia-associated lesion or mass; can be found in the colon during surveillance colonoscopy in ulcerative colitis and Crohn's colitis; associated with high probability of concurrent cancer.

Deep venous thrombosis (DVT): Blood clots that form in veins deep below the skin surface; most commonly occurs in the legs, but can occur throughout the body

Dermatitis: Skin irritation or inflammation; in IBD it often occurs around the anus.

Dermatitis herpetiformis (DH): The rash associated with celiac sprue; caused by sensitivity to gluten.

Diabetes: Elevated blood sugar (glucose).

Distention: Abdominal bloating usually from excess amounts of gas in the intestines; can be a sign of a bowel obstruction.

Diverticulitis: Inflammation or infection of a diverticulum; symptoms can mimic Crohn's disease.

Diverticulosis: A disorder characterized by small outpouchings of the colon that commonly develop as you age; a diverticulum can become infected (causing diverticulitis) and can hemorrhage.

Dysplasia: A premalignant cellular change seen on biopsy prior to the development of cancer; can occur in the colon in ulcerative colitis or Crohn's colitis, but can also be found in other organs not related to IBD, such as cervical dysplasia (which is what a pap smear examines for) or esophageal dysplasia in Barrett's esophagus.

Enteroclysis: A radiologic examination that provides a detailed examination of the small bowel. A small tube is passed through the nose, into the stomach, and out into the duodenum;

barium is then instilled through the tube directly into the small bowel. This is an excellent test to detect small abnormalities in the small intestine that may not have been detected on a small bowel follow-through.

Episcleritis: Inflammation of the whites of the eye; can occur in IBD.

Episiotomy: An incision made in the vaginal wall during childbirth to prevent a vaginal tear.

ERCP: Endoscopic retrograde cholangiopancteatography; this is an endoscopic procedure used to examine the bile duct and the pancreatic duct. This procedure is performed for a variety of reasons, including to detect and remove stones in the common bile duct, to detect tumors involving the bile or pancreatic ducts, and to diagnose primary sclerosing cholangitis.

Erythema nodosum: A red, painful swelling that can occur on the legs and arms in patients with IBD; can also be associated with other diseases.

EUA (evaluation under anesthesia): Physical examination of the rectum and perirectal area performed when the patient is anesthetized; usually done to evaluate for an abscess and/or fistula. An EUA is often performed to allow the surgeon to drain the abscess and place a Seton (drainage tube).

Exacerbation: An increase in the activity of disease; a flare.

Extraintestinal manifestations: Signs of IBD that are found outside of the gastrointestinal tract, hence the term *extraintestinal.*

Familial polyposis: An inherited, premalignant condition in which the colon is lined with hundreds of polyps.

FDA: Food and Drug Administration; the federal agency that is primarily responsible for overseeing the nation's drug approval process and for monitoring drug safety.

Fissure: A crack or split, which, in IBD, most often occurs in the anal canal.

Fistula: A tunnel connecting two structures that are not normally connected; examples include a fistula between the rectum and vagina (rectovaginal fistula) or the colon and bladder (colovesicular fistula).

Flatus: Gas passed per rectum.

Food allergy: An immune system response to a food that the body mistakenly believes is harmful.

Food intolerance: An adverse reaction to food that does not involve the immune system.

Gallbladder: A small sack adjacent to the liver where bile is stored.

Gallstones: Stones that form in the gallbladder.

Gastritis: Inflammation of the stomach.

Gastroenteritis: An intestinal illness characterized by abdominal cramps and diarrhea; usually caused by an infection.

Gastroenterologist: A physician who specializes in diseases of the gastrointestinal tract, liver, and pancreas.

Gastroenterology: The study of diseases of the digestive system. Physicians who treat IBD specialize in the field of gastroenterology.

Gastrointestinal tract: The digestive tube that starts at the mouth and ends at the anus.

General anesthesia: A form of deep sedation in which patients are given medicines to induce a state of unresponsiveness; patients under general anesthesia do not feel even painful stimuli.

Genetic predisposition: An inherited trait that makes one more likely to develop a disease.

Giardiasis: Intestinal infection with the parasite *Giardia*; commonly causes cramps and diarrhea.

Gingivitis: Inflammation of the gums.

Glaucoma: Increased pressure within the eye.

Gluten: A protein found in wheat, rye, barley, and sometimes oats; exposure to this protein causes celiac sprue in susceptible individuals.

Gluten-free diet: The diet followed by individuals with celiac sprue in which only food that does not contain gluten can be eaten.

Granuloma: A certain type of cell found in Crohn's disease; can also be seen in other, nongastrointestinal diseases.

Granulomatous colitis: Crohn's disease of the colon.

Granulomatous enteritis: Crohn's disease of the small bowel.

Gout: Type of arthritis characterized by uric acid crystal deposition in the joints; often presents as a red, swollen, painful big toe.

Hemorrhage: Abnormally heavy bleeding.

Hemorrhagic colitis: Colitis that has been complicated by severe bleeding. Hemorrhagic colitis can develop in patients with severe ulcerative colitis.

Hemorrhoids: Engorged veins found around the anus that are commonly found in IBD patients. Often they bleed and can cause rectal pain if blood becomes clotted within the hemorrhoids, which is a condition called thrombosed hemorrhoids.

Hydrogen breath test: A test to diagnose bacterial overgrowth.

Hydronephrosis: Fluid retention in the kidneys caused by obstruction of the ureter (the tube that connects the kidneys to the bladder); most commonly a result of kidney stones that have slipped into the ureter, but can also occur in the setting of severe Crohn's disease in which swelling of the bowel impinges on the ureter.

Hypertension: High blood pressure.

Ileal pouch anal anastomosis: Operation performed mostly in ulcerative colitis in which part of the ileum is used to construct an internal pouch that is connected to the anus.

Ileitis: Inflammation of the ileum; old term for Crohn's disease that is now infrequently used. Ileal inflammation can have causes other than Crohn's disease, such as infection. Individuals with Crohn's disease of the ileum are said to have ileitis.

Ileostomy: A surgically created connection between the intestine and the skin to allow for the diversion of fecal material; the waste empties into a bag attached to the skin.

Immune dysregulation: Failure of the body to appropriately regulate the immune system; this lack or regulation is believed to be integral to the development of Crohn's disease and ulcerative colitis.

Immune modulators: A class of drugs that modulates or suppresses the immune system.

Immune system: An internal network of organs, cells, and structures that work to guard your body against foreign substances, such as infections.

Immunology: The study of the immune system.

Incontinence: Leakage of stool (fecal incontinence) or urine (urinary incontinence) as a result of a loss of control.

Induction of remission: Term used to describe the use of drug therapy to treat active symptoms and bring about a remission.

Inflammation: A process characterized by swelling, warmth, redness, and/or tenderness; can occur in any organ.

INR: A blood test used to monitor warfarin sodium (Coumadin) therapy.

Intestinal stasis: The condition in which fluid no longer flows freely through the intestinal tract, usually due to a blockage; can lead to bacterial overgrowth.

Iritis: Inflammation of the iris, which is the colored part of the eye. Can occur in IBD.

Irritable bowel syndrome (IBS): A functional disorder characterized by atypical abdominal pain, diarrhea, constipation, diarrhea alternating with constipation, the feeling of incomplete fecal evacuation, or any combination of these symptoms.

J-pouch: Same as an ileal pouch anal anastomosis; the J-pouch is named as such because the pouch is constructed in the shape of the letter *J*.

Jaundice: Yellowing of the skin and whites of the eyes; usually a result of liver disease.

Kidney stones: Stones that form in the kidneys.

Lactase: The intestinal enzyme responsible for the breakdown of lactose; deficiency in this enzyme leads to lactose malabsorption.

Lactose breath test: A test used to diagnose intolerance to lactose.

Lactose intolerance: The inability to absorb dairy products caused by a deficiency of the lactase enzyme; a type of malabsorption disorder.

Latent tuberculosis: This term refers to a tuberculosis infection that is dormant (inactive infection).

Left-sided colitis: Ulcerative colitis that involves the left side of the colon.

Liver fibrosis: Scar tissue in the liver, usually from prior inflammation.

Lymphoma: Cancer of the lymphatic system, that is, the lymph nodes.

Maintenance of remission: The term used to describe the use of drug therapy to maintain a patient in remission.

Malabsorption: A condition in which the small intestine is not able to absorb nutrients and vitamins.

Malignancy: Cancer.

Malnutrition: A condition in which your body has not taken in enough nutrients and vitamins to maintain good health.

Melena: A bowel movement composed of dark, tarry stool; indicates bleeding from the upper gastrointestinal tract.

Mesenteric ischemia: Loss of blood flow to the intestines.

MRI: Magnetic resonance imaging; a radiologic examination that uses a magnetic field to create a detailed picture of structures and organs within the body. An MRI is especially helpful in detecting abdominal and pelvic abscesses.

Mucosa: The innermost lining of the intestines.

Nasogastric suction: A long, flexible tube that is passed through the nose into the stomach and is used to suction out the stomach in the setting of a bowel obstruction or sometimes after an operation.

NSAID: Nonsteroidal anti-inflammatory drug; anti-inflammatory medication commonly used to treat headaches and joint and muscle aches.

NSAID enterocolopathy: Ulcers throughout the small bowel and colon caused by the use of NSAIDs.

Obstruction: A blockage of the small intestine or colon.

Ocular: Refers to the eye.

Osteoarthritis: Arthritis caused by natural wear and tear on the joints; commonly occurs in older individuals, but can also be found in younger athletes as a result of years of trauma.

Osteonecrosis: Also called avascular necrosis; severe deterioration of the bone. It can occur after long-term use of corticosteroids and is usually diagnosed by an MRI of the affected joint.

Osteopenia: A mild decrease in bone density; can occur after long-term use of corticosteroids.

Osteoporosis: A severe decrease in bone density; can occur after long-term use of corticosteroids.

Ostomy: Same as stoma.

Pancolitis: Extensive ulcerative colitis; ulcerative colitis that extends beyond the left colon.

Pancreas: An abdominal organ with dual functions; it is a digestive organ that produces enzymes to aid in the digestion of protein, fats, and carbohydrates, and it is also an endocrine organ that produces insulin.

Pancreatitis: Inflammation of the pancreas; most often caused by gallstones, alcohol use, or as a drug side effect.

Pathergy phenomenon: An unusual dermatologic condition that occurs in pyoderma gangrenosum, in which even minor trauma can cause a skin ulcer to become bigger.

Pathologist: A physician trained in the evaluation of organs, tissues, and cells, usually under a microscope; assists in determining and characterizing the presence of disease.

Peptic ulcer disease: The condition in which an ulcer forms in the stomach or duodenum; may be from acid or the bacteria *Helicobacter pylori.*

Perforation: A rupture or abnormal opening of the intestine that allows intestinal contents to escape into the abdominal cavity.

Perianal: The area adjacent to the outside of the anus; common site for abscess and fistula formation.

Peritonitis: Inflammation or infection of the peritoneum; this is a common complication of a perforation.

PMS: premenstrual syndrome; a mood change, sometimes dramatic, that can be seen in some women just prior to the start of menstruation.

Polyp: Small, benign growth commonly found in the colon and less commonly found elsewhere in the gastrointestinal tract.

Pouchitis: Inflammation of the ileal pouch.

Prednisone-dependent: A term used to describe an individual who responds to prednisone but has a flare upon tapering.

Prednisone-refractory: A term used to describe an individual who does not respond to prednisone.

Prednisone-withdrawal syndrome: A constellation of symptoms that includes fatigue, lethargy, lassitude, and muscle and joint aches that can occur after stopping prednisone.

Prevalence: The number of people affected by a disease in a population at a specific time.

Primary sclerosing cholangitis (PSC): Inflammation and scarring of the bile ducts within the liver; can occur in IBD.

Probiotics: Healthy bacteria that can be ingested with the goal of repopulating the digestive system with "good" bacteria.

Proctectomy: Surgical removal of the rectum. Individuals with Crohn's colitis or ulcerative colitis sometimes need to have a protectomy.

Proctitis: Inflammation of the rectum.

Proctocolectomy: Surgical removal of the rectum and colon.

Proctoscopy: A procedure in which a rigid, straight, lighted tube is used to examine the rectum; usually this examination is performed on a special tilt table that positions the patient with the head down and buttocks up. Although this procedure has mostly been replaced by flexible sigmoidoscopy, it is still an excellent test to examine the rectum.

Proctosigmoiditis: Inflammation of the rectum and sigmoid colon.

Prolapsed ostomy: When the ostomy sticks out more than usual.

Prophylactic colectomy: Removal of the colon to prevent colon cancer from developing; performed in the case of familial polyposis. Prophylactic colectomy used to be the standard of care for long-standing ulcerative colitis, but since the advent of colonoscopy with surveillance biopsies, it is not commonly recommended.

Prophylactic therapy: Term that refers to the use of medication to prevent something from occurring, such as drug therapy after a resection for Crohn's disease to prevent the Crohn's disease from recurring.

Pruritus: Itching.

Psoriasis: A type of chronic skin inflammation.

PT (prothrombin time): A blood test used to monitor warfarin sodium (Coumadin) therapy.

Pulmonary embolus (PE): A blood clot that has traveled to the lungs.

Pyoderma gangrenosum: A skin ulcer that can occur in IBD patients anywhere on the skin, but most commonly is found on the extremities and immediately adjacent to a stoma.

Pyostomatitis vegetans: A rare oral form of Crohn's disease in which multiple, small pustules, ulcers, and abscesses develop in the oral cavity.

Recurrence: The reappearance of a disease.

Regional enteritis: Same as small bowel Crohn's disease; this is an old term that is now used infrequently.

Remission: The state of having no active disease. It can refer to clinical remission, meaning no symptoms are present; endoscopic remission, meaning no disease is detected endoscopically; or histologic remission, meaning no active inflammation is detected on biopsy.

Resection: The surgical removal of a segment of intestine.

Restorative proctocolectomy: Another name for an ileal pouch anal anastomosis.

Rheumatoid arthritis: A type of chronic joint inflammation.

Risk: The chance or probability that something will or will not happen.

Risk factor: Factors that predispose a person to getting a disease; for example, smoking is a risk factor for lung cancer.

Sedation: Also called conscious sedation, or moderate sedation; sedation is a form of moderate anesthesia in which the patient is given medication to induce a state of relaxation. Patients under sedation are sleepy and are less likely to feel discomfort.

Sepsis: Severe infection that spreads through the bloodstream.

Seton: A small, thin, flexible piece of tubing that is inserted through the skin, into an abscess, out of the abscess, into the rectum, and then out through the anus where the two ends are tied together. A Seton is placed to prevent an abscess from re-forming or a fistula from closing.

Short gut syndrome: A condition of severe malabsorption caused by extensive small bowel resection.

Sickle cell anemia: Inherited blood disorder that can cause anemia.

Side effect: An adverse reaction to a medication or treatment.

Sigmoidoscopy: This procedure is basically a "short" colonoscopy and is used to examine the rectum and left colon.

Sign: Objective evidence of disease; a characteristic that can be identified on physical examination or by a test.

Skin tag: A piece of excess anal or perianal tissue that hangs off the anus.

Somnolence: The state of sleepiness or drowsiness.

Specific carbohydrate diet: A grain-free, lactose-free, sucrose-free diet that purportedly is beneficial in Crohn's disease and ulcerative colitis; a paucity of scientific evidence supports this claim.

Statistical significance: A term that means the results reported in a scientific study (i.e., an experiment) are probably true and did not occur by chance.

Steroid: Another name for corticosteroid; a potent anti-inflammatory drug.

Stoma: The surgically created opening where the intestine or colon meets the skin in an ileostomy or colostomy, respectively.

Stricture: A narrowed area of intestine usually caused by scar tissue.

Strictureplasty: An operation to open up an intestinal stricture.

Surgeon: A doctor who is trained to perform an operation.

Symptom: Subjective evidence for the existence of a disease.

Systemic: A process that involves the whole body, as opposed to a localized process; for example, fatigue is a systemic symptom, whereas lower back pain is a local symptom.

T score: A measurement of bone density in which the patient's bone density is compared to that of a young healthy adult who has excellent bone density.

Tenesmus: Intense rectal spasm, usually caused by inflammation.

Thalassemia: Inherited blood disorder that can cause anemia.

Thrombophlebitis: Inflamed superficial vein in the skin caused by a blood clot.

Thrombosed hemorrhoid: When blood clots within a hemorrhoid, the hemorrhoid is said to be thrombosed; can cause rectal pain.

Thrombosis: Blood clot.

Thrush: Oral (mouth and throat) fungal infection; appears as a whitish plaque on the tongue and on the inside lining of the mouth.

TNF: Tumor necrosis factor; this protein plays a central role in the initiation of inflammation in IBD. First described in the setting of tumors, we now know that TNF is commonly found in many inflammatory conditions.

Topical therapy: A type of therapy that is applied directly to tissue; commonly used in inflammation of the rectum and left colon.

Toxic megacolon: Acute distention with air of the colon that usually occurs in the setting of severe colitis; can occur in Crohn's colitis, ulcerative colitis, or infectious colitis.

TPN (total parenteral nutrition): Nutrition supplied intravenously.

Tuberculosis: An infection with *Mycobacterium tuberculosis*.

Tumor: An abnormal growth of tissue; can be benign or malignant.

Ulcerative colitis: A disease characterized by chronic inflammation of the colon.

Ultrasound: A radiologic study that uses sound waves to examine abdominal and pelvic organs; commonly used to look for gallstones and obstruction of the bile duct.

Upper endoscopy: A procedure in which a small, thin, flexible, lighted tube with a camera on the end is passed through the mouth into the esophagus, stomach, and duodenum; an excellent test to detect inflammation and strictures in the upper gastrointestinal tract that allows a biopsy to be taken.

Upper GI series/upper GI series with small bowel follow-through: A radiologic examination of the esophagus, stomach, duodenum, and small bowel. The patient drinks a thick, white liquid shake of barium, and then the barium is tracked by taking X rays as it travels through the gastrointestinal tract. This is an excellent test to detect strictures, fistulas, and inflammation in the stomach and small bowel.

Ureter: The tube that connects the kidneys to the bladder and through which urine flows.

Urethra: The tunnel that connects the bladder to the outside of the body through which urine passes.

Urgency: The feeling that you have to move your bowels or urinate right away.

Uveitis: Inflammation of the uvea, which is the central part of the eye (the iris is part of the uvea); can occur in IBD.

Virtual colonoscopy: A CT scan of the colon; this radiologic study is still in early development but shows promise as a method to detect colonic abnormalities.

X ray: A radiologic study that provides an image of bodily structures.

Z score: A measurement of bone density in which the patient's bone density is compared to the bone density of a person of the same age, gender, and race.

Index